FLEX MOM

Advance Praise

"*Flex Mom* gives you permission, and teaches you to give yourself permission, to invest in your own well-being. It can actually help you become a happier and better parent."

—**Dr. Tal Ben-Shahar**, author of *Happier*
and co-founder of Potentialife

"*Flex Mom* honors the complexities of motherhood today and provides thoughtful, practical, and compassionate reflection and insight—along with a bit of humor. Blanchard's honesty and perspective paves the way for exploring this third dimension of parenting, and seeks to support the reader along her journey. Whether you are ready to launch into being a Flex Mom today or just exploring what might be possible in the future, this book is for you."

—**Sarah**, PhD and proud Flex Mom

"It was an a-ha kind of moment, opening these pages—this type of motherhood has been in the universe, but until Sara Blanchard put it into words, I didn't know it existed. If it weren't for *Flex Mom*, I wouldn't have the balance to follow my passion as an author and still be the mom who picks up her kids after school."

—**Erin Lockwood**, author of *Planning Penelope*

"I loved this book! The author writes with such personal insight and humor about the joys and struggles of being a stay-at-home mom—I found myself nodding along throughout the whole book. Any mom who stays at home can benefit from reading this and thinking about how she can incorporate the ideas of being a Flex Mom into her life."

—**Emily**, former cosmetics executive, now stay-at-home mom in NYC

"Smart, unique and easy to implement, this book is written for the woman who is ready to shift from unhappy and unchallenged at home, to being excited about raising kids and pursuing her own passions. There are so many great ideas for a happy life in this book, I recommend it for working moms too!"

—**Jaime Myers**, owner of Shine Life Design

"There's so much more work to staying at home than there was in my generation. My children were always active, but it was usually stuff they did on their own; now there is so much parental involvement in playdates and sports leagues. Add that to what seems like pressure for moms to make a financial contribution or to have an identity outside of the house, and I can see where moms now seem less happy than I remember my generation feeling. *Flex Mom* helps bridge that gap, to help moms get back to the core of what they want to provide for their families and regain a sense of self."

—**Bonnie**, former stay-at-home mom, now grandmother

FLEX MOM

THE SECRETS OF HAPPY STAY-AT-HOME MOMS

SARA BLANCHARD

NEW YORK

NASHVILLE • MELBOURNE • VANCOUVER

FLEX MOM
THE SECRETS OF HAPPY STAY-AT-HOME MOMS

© 2017 **SARA BLANCHARD**

Published in New York, New York, by Morgan James Publishing in partnership with Difference Press. Morgan James is a trademark of Morgan James, LLC. www.MorganJamesPublishing.com

The Morgan James Speakers Group can bring authors to your live event. For more information or to book an event visit The Morgan James Speakers Group at www.TheMorganJamesSpeakersGroup.com.

ISBN 978-1-68350-559-4 paperback
ISBN 978-1-68350-560-0 eBook
Library of Congress Control Number: 2017906586

Cover Design by:
Rachel Lopez
www.r2cdesign.com

Interior Design by:
Bonnie Bushman
The Whole Caboodle Graphic Design

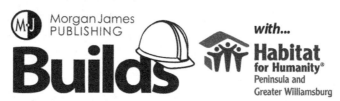

In an effort to support local communities, raise awareness and funds, Morgan James Publishing donates a percentage of all book sales for the life of each book to Habitat for Humanity Peninsula and Greater Williamsburg.

Get involved today! Visit
www.MorganJamesBuilds.com

DEDICATION

To my daughters, Cassady and Annika.
For you, I work to find a better way.

TABLE OF CONTENTS

FOREWORD

My freshmen year at Harvard, I overheard two people talking about a woman who had graduated a few years ago and had left her job at a private equity firm to stay home with her kids. One of the guys sneered, "Isn't she a little overqualified for that?" I am still upset today thinking about the ignorance of that statement and the stigma on parents who deviate from the reckless pursuit of a narrowly defined type of productivity. This is not just a question of maternity or paternity leave for parents in the first few months of a new baby. This is an issue which makes us question how to live a valuable life, why work is meaningful, when to leave work in the day, whether we take vacations, and whether we should turn to "productive" emails after hours or on the weekend.

When Sara and I sat down to a meal in the spring of 2008, it was not at a lavish restaurant befitting young professional colleagues, but at a dorm dining hall surrounded by chatty, boisterous undergrads. We were in the midst of teaching sections for Harvard's most popular course—

Positive Psychology 1504—and I was drafting my book *The Happiness Advantage*. In the midst of a monochromatic dining hall meal we spoke about the ripple effect, about the thrills and difficulties of book writing and life coaching, and about how we couldn't wait for the next time all of us teaching fellows would head out to get "real food," which basically meant not eating on a tray. Who knew that despite all of our plans for consulting and research and the future of positive psychology, in the near future, Sara and her husband would soon have a child, and she would leave the workforce. And she was not alone.

Consider the statistics. Data released by the Centers for Disease Control and Prevention showed an increasing number of American women—now over 30%—are waiting until their 30s to have their first child. Mothers in this country are having children later in life, meaning they've had a taste of working, of having a career, before they add the new title of parent onto their resume. I have witnessed how challenging it is to give up a blossoming career to focus entirely on someone else. And, there are millions of people in this country who do it all the time. Of the roughly 34 million families with children under 18, both parents worked in roughly 60% of those families. Even conservatively, if we say that half of those parents who didn't work, did not work by choice, that would mean at least 7 million parents have chosen to stay at home to raise their children. There are millions of parents who are struggling with the "in-between," wanting to continue their own personal trajectory while also wanting to prioritize their children. It's a question I ask every day as I structure my day or think about traveling for work. But due to the nature of our biology, this question often weighs heavier among our moms.

My wife, Michelle Gielan, lives the lifestyle Sara describes in *Flex Mom*, even though we didn't have a name for it when we started. This new model of parenthood, Flex Mom—the third model that sits somewhere between stay-at-home moms and working moms—is one that Michelle has operated by ever since we had our first child. She and I met first as colleagues, researching and spreading happiness together, and with her magnetic personality and brilliant mind, I wouldn't have wanted her to feel like she had to give up that side of herself to raise our son Leo. Yet, our child means the world to us and with our hectic travel schedules, we wouldn't have wanted to leave him at home to be raised by anybody but us. We created the space in our lives to give our son the love he needs, while continuing to work to spread the happiness that brought us together as a family in the first place. And it has been both a sacrifice and a joy.

Everyone's path is different, but in this book is a clearly outlined path of transformation from stay-at-home mom to Flex Mom. Sara arms you with the skills and structures you need to clear the space to pursue your passion, while continuing to be the primary caregiver for your children. She incorporates well-researched methods like mindfulness and goal-setting, and melds those into the daily struggles that people with children know so well.

Sara is the real deal. She is incredibly intelligent and capable, while being humble and compassionate. With Sara's extensive experience in positive psychology, both through life coaching and teaching the course at Harvard, and her background of transition from corporate America to stay-at-home motherhood, it seems only fitting that she has identified a way to help other women who have had to consciously shift their thoughts about careers and parenting. I am thrilled that she is helping other mothers find ways to prioritize their children while creating space to pursue their own goals. Flex Mom is a powerful model and has the potential to lift women up in a world which is in desperate need of their leadership, their wisdom, and their happiness.

—**Shawn Achor**, *New York Times* bestselling author of
The Happiness Advantage

THE LOST LUCKY ONES

"I think it's a tough road if you're a stay-at-home mom, a working mom, if you have a partner, if you don't. It's the best job in the world, and the toughest job in the world all at the same time."
—Angela Kinsey

Since the second wave of feminism in the 1960s challenged the notion of women as homemakers, we have come to loosely accept the idea that strong, powerful women should compete in the workforce with men. While there is still plenty of room for improvement in pay equality, opportunities, and ultimately, in breaking the glass ceiling, this and subsequent feminist movements have given rise to career women. When career women bore children, these movements allowed for them to become working moms. While earlier in history the stay-at-home mom (SAHM) was the norm, it is now much more common for children to have working moms. Given this background, when you have children now, there are two models of motherhood to choose between: working mom or stay-at-home mom.

This book is for mothers who have the financial bandwidth and have chosen to be the primary caregivers for their children. While much of the following reading will be helpful to working mothers, I cannot speak with expertise on the experience of being a traditional working mom with an office job—and more importantly, I cannot help you calculate the numbers to make it feasible for you to take a step back from the money. But, if you can work out your financials so that you are not totally dependent on your salary and you decide to become the primary caregiver for your children, then this book is absolutely for you.

I recently met Genevieve, who has a PhD in microbiology and enjoyed her career in cancer research. She and her husband moved around quite a bit as his career grew, but she was always able to find a position doing the work she loved. Enter children. A couple of years into parenthood, the 60 hour workweeks became significantly overwhelming, and the job she enjoyed became a burden as she struggled with being away from her little ones for so long. Barely able to juggle her work life and home life, Genevieve left her job—preserving great relationships with her bosses who said they'd welcome her back anytime—and greatly appreciated that she was able to stay at home. The first few months of being able to focus solely on her children were wonderful, and Genevieve filled the time with books and games and outings to the library. But less than a year into staying at home, she started feeling isolated and lonely, underappreciated and undervalued. The novelty of interacting with her small children wore off, and she found herself craving conversations with her colleagues, wanting to make contributions to the greater community like she did with her cancer research. Still, even though Genevieve's bosses said that she could come back part time, she knew that she would be hard pressed to find a balance she was comfortable with in her old field. While going back to her previous career wasn't the right fit, Genevieve knew she couldn't continue staying at home the way she was feeling. She started looking for something that fit her interests— somewhere between staying at home and working. If this is you, *Flex Mom* is the book you need.

The reason *Flex Mom* is for you is because it presents a third model for motherhood, a model outside of the stay-at-home vs. working mom dichotomy. This book captures the unexpected pitfalls that are unique to the stay-at-home parenting experience, and transitions you into a new way of thinking and being. Because if you've been at home with your children, I bet that at one time or another, you've thought that being a stay-at-home mom is the most difficult thing you've ever done. I certainly have thought it. I also bet that your old career, the one you had prior to children, provided you with money, prestige, and/or a sense of purpose; I bet that while that job was challenging, being with the children 24/7 has left you more depleted than your job used to. Mostly, I bet that you wish there was a way to make this supposedly amazing experience more fulfilling.

Once you have children, life changes. No matter who it is, someone has to be responsible for the little ones—and there are tons of reasons to choose to be that person who is the primary caregiver for your children. Supporters say there's no substitute for the consistency and nurturing of parental care; you worked hard to have this child, and you want to be around to help raise him or her. There are so many additional reasons to be the stay-at-home parent: maybe you hated your career and this was a natural move to make. Maybe your spouse travels for work and you would have gone nuts if you'd continued working while holding down the fort. Maybe you'd always dreamed that you'd get to stay at home, just like your own mother did. For one reason or another, you and your partner made the decision for you to be a stay-at-home mom, and because everyone tells you what a privilege it is, you expected it to be awesome.

It sure has been awesome. And awesomely difficult.

Once you made it through the sleepless survival stage of the first year, you thought things would improve. Because really, what could be worse than your colicky child screaming for a few hours at a time, and then waking up every three hours for food, for months? You took on all the overnight shifts yourself because you were the stay-at-home parent, the one who didn't have an outside responsibility to wake up for the next day. So, even though you didn't get more than one complete sleep cycle per night for months, you pushed through the fatigue and eagerly waited for the next stage.

Then you realized the toddler years were tough in a different way, with your physical exhaustion shifting to one that took over more of your brain. You read the same books over and over again, shell shocked by the mind-numbing repetition that comes with young children. You fought the urge to put on Baby Einstein DVDs because, even though you wanted a break from the (cute) monotony, you felt guilty after the latest round of research showed that the DVDs didn't really improve cognitive skills. You had to interpret your child's grunts and squeals, figuring out which one meant hungry and which one meant they wanted to grab your fingers so they could waddle-walk with your hunched-over help. Surely, you thought, once your child started speaking in sentences and could navigate a playground without your help, child rearing would be more joyful and fulfilling.

By the time your children entered preschool, though, you found that you were so tired from giving and giving and giving that you didn't even know where to start to fill your own bucket again, where to find the energy to play and be joyful again.

The double edged sword for stay-at-home moms in middle- or upper-class families is that, for this particular crust of society, sociologist Annette Lareau observed that children are seen as projects to be cultivated. Unlike past generations, whose main goals were to feed the kids and keep them alive with the expectation that the kids would turn out okay, our generation gets a kick out of intentional parenting. As exhausting as it is to answer each question and nurture each talent, few parents want to neglect this work because they're afraid of not giving their child every advantage possible. Even though it's draining to focus so much on parenting your children, you do it anyway.

You're not alone in finding parenting difficult. A study by behavioral economist Daniel Kahneman showed—unwittingly—that when women were asked to rate activities that gave them the most pleasure, childcare was very low on the list. These parents would have preferred shopping, watching TV, and even preparing food and vacuuming to taking care of children. And I totally hate vacuuming. Still, while it's nice to know you're not alone—and you probably got a glimpse of this commonality as you met eyes across the playground with the other exhausted moms, then rolling those eyes in sympathy with each other—it doesn't help point you in the right direction to take a step towards actually enjoying your life as a stay-at-home parent.

The thing is, it's not cool to complain about the privilege of staying at home. We are considered the lucky ones, the ones who have enough money, who "only" have the responsibility of raising children; working moms have to do it all while juggling a real career.

And it's true—we really are lucky to be in a financial position that our partner can support our living expenses and those of our children. It's a luxury that not everybody in this country has, and there are many working moms who would love to be able to stay home to raise their children instead of having to work to support the family's financial needs. Statistics from 2015 show that among married-couple families with children, 60% of these families had both parents working; that means that it's the minority, or 40%, of families who have one unemployed parent, whether by choice or by circumstance. What frustrated stay-at-home parents want to share, though, is that it's not just a happy-go-lucky lifestyle that we live. The freedom not to work comes with its own set of burdens. What people don't see is that you probably left a major metropolitan area to live somewhere less expensive so your family could afford this lifestyle. They don't see the deliberation that goes into each pedicure or new item of clothing that you buy for yourself—the guilt that, annoyingly, you don't seem to have when spending money on your children's enrichment classes, or that your partner doesn't seem to have when buying some new gadgets for the home. Most of the time, the stay-at-home parenting lifestyle was created by design, after reflecting on family values, individual values, and financial capacity. It's not just luck. There is a lot of work that goes into this choice, and work that goes into making it through each day.

Outside observers don't see that kids make huge messes when they're home instead of at daycare, so you don't get to take naps when they are sleeping because you're busy returning your house to normal. They don't see that it's mind-numbing to listen to imaginary stories all day, to not have the mental stimulation that the give-and-take of adult conversation provides. They don't see that you don't get a lunch break, that you never get a sick day, that you don't have time for yourself until bedtime, and that you love your children dearly but can't wait to get away from them. They don't see that you can't say any of these things to outsiders, because then you'd sound like you're complaining. So the bulk of stay-at-home moms live in quiet guilt. And the guilt grows until you feel like a shell of yourself, and your sense of purpose is lost.

Fortunately, there is hope: being the primary caregiver for your children doesn't have to make you feel so invisible and lonely. This book draws upon my years of being a miserable stay-at-home mom with a passion for and former career in mind-body wellness—one who finally figured out through trial and error what it takes to make this time raising my children a more fulfilling experience.

The new name for a thriving, caregiving parent is the Flex Mom. The Flex Mom continues to prioritize her children, but understands how to create the space and structure to pursue her own passions. She sets goals outside of her family life—goals that fuel her passions and fit within the lifestyle she wants to live—while continuing to be present with her children in the same way that stay-at-home parents are. The Flex Mom flows between multiple roles, and the energy she gets from being lit up with excitement about pursuing her goals fuels back into her home life. This book outlines the steps you need to take to make the transformation.

While there are lots of stories and theories to learn from in *Flex Mom*, scattered through these pages are also some exercises to help you make changes in your life as you go. If you want to skip over those and simply read through, you should still be able to follow along. If you want to do the exercises, check the back of the book to learn how to get a free companion workbook that will help you process your thoughts as you work through these pages.

The steps to becoming a Flex Mom are:

F: Free yourself from judgment, because you are probably your own worst critic

L: Love yourself, and learn how to take care of yourself first

E: Express your goals, goals that are in line with your skills and passions and mean something to you

X: Examine your boundaries and community to carve out space so you can achieve your goals

M: Master skills around mindfulness, because just as you think you've got things figured out, things will change—and mindfulness will let you see your options

O: Open your mouth wisely and master crucial communication skills to get what you want

M: Make it all come together

There are many, many benefits to being a stay-at-home parent, to being able to hold space for your children and your household. However, being miserable during the experience negates some of these benefits for your children, and leaves you feeling like you've spent several years of your life floundering around. This book is intended to help you nip that misery in the bud before you squander any more of these precious childhood years. By learning how to hold space not only for your family, but for your own personal goals and passions, you'll join the ranks of Flex Moms—moms who continue to be present for their children in the same way stay-at-home parents are, but who are energized by pursuing the things they want to be doing.

CHAPTER 1
NOTES FROM A MISERABLE SAHM

"With what price we pay for the glory of motherhood."
—Isadora Duncan

S traight after graduating from Harvard, I started my career at Goldman Sachs and joined the ranks of the successful young professional, living in Tokyo and Hong Kong, working hard and playing hard. Several years into this life, my dad—my closest confidant—suddenly passed away and I found myself reevaluating my priorities. Knowing that he'd always told me to "keep the balance," I eventually found an even more fulfilling career working as a life coach and focusing on positive psychology. I even helped teach Harvard's most popular undergraduate course, where I met inspiring people who wanted to help the world get happier. I thought that, unlike finance, this would be the career I'd be able to continue when I had kids, because I got to design my own hours and, c'mon, it was focused on people being HAPPY, for crying out loud. I could do that while parenting.

Then, my first child was born. She is an old soul, wise beyond her years. Unfortunately, being aware of so much while so young, she worried loads about her daddy's absence when he traveled for work, and didn't seem to understand that I was always going to be around at nighttime. My daughter became super dependent on my presence. On top of these attachment issues, she developed GI issues and sleep issues, and I couldn't find a consistent hour for a coaching call with my clients without her screams emanating from the other side of the house. The sitter would try to calm her, but she'd cry, my boobs would start streaming breast milk, and I'd be distracted. It wasn't fair to my clients, to my child, or to me. So, reluctantly, with the support of my husband, who saw me slowly fading with the conflict, I shuttered my coaching business indefinitely.

It wasn't an easy choice. My mom had stayed at home with me until I left for college, so it's fair to say that I'd had that option in the back of my mind. I had also consciously made the transition out of finance and its 14-hour workdays to a more balanced life coaching practice with an eye on a flexible lifestyle, so I knew that in my heart, having children and being present for them was a priority for me. Still, I'd left the Ivy League and Wall Street labels behind—and now that parenting was my full time gig, I wasn't sure how to judge myself against any metrics of success. I kept reading about my old colleagues' successes. I heard about their new financial milestones, and wondered if I'd made the right choice. I wasn't counting clients, money earned, or emails sent, and as far as I'd found, there was no way to know if I was doing well at this new "job." I wished for a crystal ball so I could see my children as adults to know whether I was turning them into monsters or angels with every seemingly major decision I made. I found myself second guessing a lot, wondering if I'd wasted my potential, and feeling a little lost about how to interact with an eight-month-old for so many hours at a time.

Then came society's judgment. After making the decision to stay at home, the first adult function I went to was a microfinance fundraiser that a close girlfriend was hosting. I put on nice clothes and mentally warmed up my social skills. Drink in hand, I mingled and shook hands, listening and asking questions and feeling good about being among peers again. A woman with a sharp haircut and black pantsuit introduced herself to me and proceeded to tell me all about how she was such an important person in Scottsdale, being a Vice President of a local bank branch up the street. With my experience working around the world at an international financial firm, I listened silently with some perspective—and then the tables turned. She asked the dreaded question, "What do you do?" and I took a deep breath, recounted the promise I made to myself not to qualify my decision, and answered, "I stay at home with my kids."

The only face I recall going blanker than hers was that of my grandfather, who'd been diagnosed with Alzheimer's and would flick in and out of awareness. She replied with an "oh," turned on her heel, and started immediately chatting with the next available person. It took all of my self-control not to shout after her, to tell her all of my past accomplishments and prove to her that I was still a person worth speaking with. I was shaking with anger, and only after a week or so did I realize that it wasn't about me—that I actually ought to feel sorry for her lack of social skills. She could have asked my children's ages, what my interests were, who I knew at the fundraiser, anything. But no amount of afterthought could erase the emotional impact that her ignorance and judgment had on me. I wasn't yet confident in my decision to stay at home, and her judgment tipped the scales to the dark side—I started feeling unworthy.

What were some of the ways I felt crappy being a SAHM? Money, guilt, resentment, invisibility—just, you know, a few minor issues.

My husband John and I earned enough money, and we purposely left the greater New York area to move to the much more affordable Phoenix / Scottsdale area in Arizona after we got married. I used to make as much as my husband in my finance days, but my coaching practice hadn't ramped up to that level again, so giving up my salary wasn't as large of an adjustment as it could have been. Still, even within the framework of having similar attitudes towards spending, and even with him knowing I wasn't a wild spender who would blow thousands of dollars on the latest designer bag, I felt like I had to be super frugal because I was no longer contributing to the family's bottom line. I had done a closet revamp when my oldest was past the leaky-boob spit-up stage to get rid of stained and ripped stuff, and I realized all I had was white and black clothing. I found a red t-shirt at Target that I thought would be good to wear for Valentine's Day, and to my husband it was a no-brainer—go buy the red t-shirt! But I felt bad about spending even that bit of money without clearing it with him and (luckily) getting his total support.

The transition for a family to go from "your money" and "my money" to "our money" is a slow one, and requires everyone to be on board in order for you, as a stay-at-home mom, to feel a sense of worth. Yet while your actual income goes to zero, your contribution to the home goes up. You've probably seen those websites that calculate your imagined worth, like the one from Salary.com that divides how much time your stay-at-home self does jobs like day care center teacher, janitor, cook, housekeeper, and chauffeur—which suggest that SAHMs are worth a base salary of $36,000 plus $78,000 in overtime, considering that we work 97 hours a week. (Working moms are worth about $67,000 plus their day job wages.) I feel grateful that my husband supported me, and my self-imposed financial struggle, but for a lot of people who have been hit over the head for years about how money rules the world (and therefore that how much money you make reflects your worth), it's a tough transition to make. I've had friends who've made the decision to stay at home, but have onboarded their lesser status from drunk husbands who mutter small comments like "Who do you think makes the money here?" when asked to help pick up toys. Hearing that would have enraged me and simultaneously made me feel so small—and I'd imagine it takes major strength and stamina to recover from blows like that when you are already faltering in your own self-worth. To state it again: your value is not tied to how much money you make, but society sure makes you feel that way.

As for guilt, I know that all moms have it. And in general, dads have it less than moms do. But stay-at-home mom guilt feels different from working mom guilt because, from what I understand, working moms want to be there for their kids and feel bad that they have to be away. SAHM guilt is the opposite—you are there for your kids and feel bad that you desperately want to get the heck away from them. I felt guilty because I hated it when my daughter cried. I had no idea what she wanted, because she just wanted ME, and I had never been touched or clung to that much in my life. In hindsight she was clearly uncomfortable, and we have found through trial and error that she has food sensitivities, but at that point she couldn't tell me what was wrong. How could I have hated it when she cried, when she was just trying to get help? Guilt. Another example: I still couldn't go to the gym even when my child was 18 months old because the in-gym daycare would page me after 10 minutes to come get my inconsolable child. I was out of shape, mentally dull, in need of a good sweat and I couldn't get it because of her—and then I looked at her innocent lovely little face and felt awful that I could possibly resent her for needing her mommy. Guilt. Then, another side of guilt kicked in because it seemed to me that the kids of working moms were much better adjusted to separation, and

I wondered if perhaps I was creating this anxious child because I didn't stick with my job when she was little. Guilt.

As for resentment, oh my. I messed this one up big time. My dear husband told me once over the kitchen island as he cleaned dishes for the millionth time that he was feeling like a glorified housekeeper. In my survival mode—with a two-and-a-half-year-old and a newborn—I rolled my eyes, thinking that I didn't have time to tell another child what to do, and that if he wanted to be more than that, then he should simply do it. In hindsight he was asking for help, saying that he wasn't being seen in our family and felt he could be replaced. But all I could do was see things from my own perspective. I was resentful that both our kids were born with sensitive stomachs, which meant that they did not sleep through the night for a full year. Which meant that, since I wasn't working and he was, and I was breastfeeding and he wasn't (our kids wouldn't take a bottle, and before you judge, know that it turns out she was sensitive to any formula that wasn't the stinky $50-a-can kind), I took the hit every single night and didn't sleep more than one sleep cycle a night for over a year. And when he would say in public that our kids were up so he was tired, I couldn't help wonder why, if he was awake anyway, he didn't offer to help. We found that a year into having a new child was a crucial time for each of us, as we both thought we were doing more for the house than the other. We regrouped and had some stripped-down, honest conversations about the State of our Union. But it got ugly there for a while.

Which leads me to why I felt invisible. I mean, sheesh, if my husband who still worked could feel invisible in the house, I sure could. I had given up my outside identity and taken on one that was defined solely by being in the house. Even skipping over those tough first few years of parenthood, when so much is dominated by lack of sleep and lack of structure, and talking only about post-toddler years, it's easy for stay-at-home moms to let themselves be consumed by the seemingly all-encompassing task of raising children. When it's your job to be with them, to challenge them, to nurture them, to teach them, to feed them, there's not much time (let alone energy) left for you to suddenly assert that you have to reach a certain deadline for a new project you came up with. When I was editor of a local mom's blog, when I ran a local women's social group, when I was ghostwriting for a content marketing firm, these things didn't seem worth prioritizing over the family because they weren't fully declared passions. On top of that, I beat myself up because I'd been a life coach; I lived and breathed positive psychology methodologies for improving our levels of happiness, and yet I wasn't feeling close to happy. I was a stay-at-home mom with things I simply dabbled in, which after long enough didn't make me feel like an interesting person, which then made me project that my husband didn't think I was an interesting person. Which didn't lead to the most fulfilling marriage or partnership. I would say that in today's society, the structure isn't there within the stay-at-home framework for moms to feel free to pursue their passions and feel like multi-dimensional human beings.

That is, unless you set yourself up to be a Flex Mom. This is how you can go from complacent and unhappy to proactive and happy, as you create a life that gives you the space you need to pursue your own goals while being present for your children.

CHAPTER 2
FLEX MOM, DEFINED

. . . .

"My mother taught me about the power of inspiration and courage, and she did it with a strength and a passion that I wish could be bottled."

—Carly Fiorina

B eing a stay-at-home mom can be a lonely prospect, but it doesn't have to be. Moms make the choice to be stay-at-home parents for many reasons, but ultimately the idea is to be present for your children in a way that you believe will best support their growth and development. Many moms are afraid to make this choice because of the isolation and mind-numbing repetition that accompanies the role of a stay-at-home mom in this day and age, especially as we have fallen into the habit of focusing on these children as projects to be cultivated instead of people to be enjoyed.

When talking with my friend Kim about the two choices of motherhood—stay-at-home mom or working mom—it occurred to her that both of those models referred to moms at a particular location. Moms are, according to tradition, either at home, or they're at work. But whether a mom is with her kids or is away from them, a mother is a mother—no matter where on the planet she is. Through this conversation, it became clear we needed to address not *where* you parent, but *how* you parent—and the Flex Mom movement was born.

The Flex Mom is the third option in the parenting model, somewhere between being a stay-at-home mom and a working mom. She is the designated adult in the family who prioritizes child care, much like a stay-at-home mother does; she is the one who attends the school functions and handles kid sick days and school pickup and the social calendar and driving around. However, the thing that the Flex Mom does differently from a stay-at-home mom is that she has learned the skills she needs to carve space in her life to run a parallel track to this repetitive child care, where she cultivates her own passion and sets goals for herself outside of the home. The difference between struggling stay-at-home parents and Flex Moms is that Flex Moms no longer feel invisible and overwhelmed, because they have connected with themselves and are ready to pursue their own goals while continuing to be present for their children.

My inspiration for this model came from my college friend Sarah. She is a super motivated, intelligent woman with a passion for education. Her husband has pursued his career with vigor since college and was on track to land his dream job when she got pregnant with their first child. While his dream job would be extraordinarily time- and energy- consuming, it would allow them to afford having her step back from her career and give their children the consistency they wanted to provide—important for them as a family, given that he was about to get really, really busy. Still, Sarah didn't let the idea of raising the children intimidate her. Ever the overachiever, she quickly got pregnant with her second child and, while raising the two children as toddlers, earned her PhD in education. This degree is just one step in the long-term vision she has for her own life, her life outside of child rearing.

Through the PhD program, Sarah hired a sitter to give herself some focus time during the day to work on her dissertation. She also worked late at night when her husband was out at meetings. She brought her children to interviews when they were home sick. As the kids have gotten older, she attends their school presentations, drives the kids to sports practice, and still cooks most meals at home. Now that she has her degree, the doors have been opened for Sarah to apply for and get funding to conduct independent studies on the quality of the local public high schools. She's doing this all while basically doing all the things that stay-at-home moms do—though she has never considered herself a true SAHM.

The difference between the Flex Mom and a "mompreneur" is that the Flex Mom follows her passion (education and policy, for Sarah) and, while it can lead to an income, she isn't doing it just to make a bit of money on the side. Being a Flex Mom involves pursuing something that reflects a core part of yourself, something that really resonates with your own interests. Sarah has the energy to move mountains to make her work happen because she loves education, loves teaching, loves doing studies (I don't get it, but she does)—she is fueled by the content of this parallel track she's created to full-time parenting. And it's totally inspiring to see.

The idea of the Flex Mom started crystallizing when Sarah made a connection for me. I had recently moved to Denver when Sarah—who knows my history as a life coach and positive psychology enthusiast—set up a meeting with the local high school. They were interested in launching an educational model that would use positive psychology as a cornerstone of their curriculum, and she suggested that I be the person to teach the educators some of the core principles. It NEVER would have occurred to me that I could do that, since I had been so used to calling myself a stay-at-home mom. Yet all I had to do was put my brain back in my head for a few hours, create a cheat sheet that I could share with the team, and hire a babysitter to watch my girls for a couple of hours while I walked down the street for the meeting. The a-ha moment hit me as I glowed with pride and satisfaction on my way home: it's possible to be flexible and do what you love, and not just live rigidly in a house-shaped box whose insides revolve around your children.

It took some time to develop a more defined understanding of what it takes to be a Flex Mom, because doing a one-off thing that lit my fire was not the same as having a parallel track to pursue my passion. It scared me to think about adding to my workload by doing more work in positive psychology all the time, even though it would have been thrilling to me, and it occurred to me that I had to consciously clear space in my life to build up the capacity to take on additional work. You don't want to start something you're passionate about and then have to quit halfway through because you got in way over your own head. So, I floated ideas by several friends who had been unknowingly living as Flex Moms, and they helped me agree on the crucial steps, structures, and skills needed to reach a sustainable level of fulfilling flexibility when pursuing your own interests.

What are these skills? It's all in the name.

F—Free Yourself from Judgment

Let go of your own tendencies to judge the SAHMs or working moms, the breastfeeding or bottle-feeding moms. You are your own worst critic, and need to free your mind to the possibility that you—and everyone else—are doing just fine.

L—Love Yourself

Not only is it okay, but it's necessary for you to take care of yourself first. It's like they say on the airplanes: in case of emergency, put your oxygen mask on first before helping those around you.

E—Express Your Goals

The missing link is that you forget to set goals outside of the house. These goals can be both big and small, but most importantly, have to be congruent with your ideal lifestyle and your passions.

X—Examine Your Boundaries

The best way to protect your newfound self-care and the pursuit of your goals is to set boundaries, including for your time and technology usage, and to build a supportive community.

M—Master Mindfulness

It's just like childrearing—you figure out how to handle a certain developmental stage and the kids enter a new one—so as things change, you can use mindfulness skills to adjust. This will help you navigate life's curveballs and distractions.

O—Open Your Mouth Wisely

When difficulties arise, you'll have the communication skills to get what you want, and you'll avoid the pitfalls that can sabotage your relationships.

M—Make It Come Together

Having learned how to carve out space to pursue your passion, you will feel energized as you go after your goals—and this energy will also magically feed back into your role as primary caregiver for your children.

The Flex Mom is a mom who strives to clear enough space in her life to pursue her own passions while being the primary caregiver for her children. She has learned about herself and what she stands for, knows how to take care of her basic needs, and no longer feels guilty about doing what she wants to do for herself. The Flex Mom has set clear goals and knows how to maintain the space to pursue her passions because she has worked on communicating wisely and being mindful about the choices she has. She feels hopeful and energized by her life as she raises her children.

CHAPTER 3
FREE YOURSELF FROM JUDGMENT

"I do know one thing about me: I don't measure myself by others' expectations or let others define my worth."
—Sonia Sotomayor

My youngest daughter was born with a love of fashion. One sunny morning in Arizona, years ago, I pulled off her pajama top and tried to put her into a striped t-shirt to start our day. My barely verbal daughter clamped her arms to her sides, vigorously shaking her head back and forth and grumbling "poka!" I kept trying to put her head through the neck of the shirt, she kept whipping her body around, ever increasing her volume, shouting "POKA!" I looked at her with exasperation, until I realized she was pointing to a different t-shirt sitting next to me. I went to grab this shirt, and her face and body relaxed, sliding right into the polka-dotted shirt.

Fast forward another few years, and this same little girl asked to take dance classes. We signed her up for a low-key ballet/tap dancing combo class, which many places offer for preschoolers. I didn't grow up in a big dance scene, so I called ahead to find out what kids were expected to wear, and I was told that, aside from needing tap shoes and ballet shoes, anything was fine. So, once a week, we started rolling into the dance class wearing some combination of child-selected outfits—a red Hello Kitty t-shirt and gigantic pink tutu, or a Princess Sophia dress-up skirt with a rainbow colored top. For a few weeks, there were other girls who also showed off their individual style, but a month in, I noticed that my daughter was the only one not wearing a muted pink or black leotard and skirt. There in front of me was my adorable independent child, proudly prancing in the middle of a class of mini ballerinas. Yet I stood in the back of the classroom, silently cringing at how mismatched her outfit was.

When, later that night, my daughter asked me if maybe we could go to the store and get her "one of those dancing outfits like the other girls had," my heart constricted. Had she picked up on the judgment I had of her, and had it somehow crushed her little independent spirit? Maybe this desire for conformity was a natural part of growing up, but I actually wanted her to keep her bold individuality, to keep her from following a crowd into trouble in her teenage years. I realized that, while I'd kept my judgment to myself and hadn't outwardly criticized her, she was already wise enough to pick up on what other people were doing and how maybe she might want to change, to conform to other's expectations.

It's somehow easier to see the impact of judgment and other's expectations on young ones, because we know they start with such innocence and independence—until external, societal expectations start to shape them. We, too, have gone through this transformation as we went from our own childhood to adulthood, and now to this stage of parenting. But how often do you step back to think about what it is that's yours, your individuality that you want to offer, versus how much you're shrinking or changing to fit what it is that others expect or want from you?

As I mentioned in the introduction to this book, I felt judged as a stay-at-home mom by a working woman I met at a fundraiser. She couldn't continue a conversation with me once she found out that I didn't have a paid job. It crushed me at first to feel like someone else thought I wasn't worthy, but the reality was, her judgment was only a reflection of my own. If I had been totally confident in my decision to be a stay-at-home mom, I wouldn't have felt the sting of her judgment. It was only because I had been judging *myself*, because I was still having doubts about the worthiness of my choice to be at home, that I felt small. This is the cycle of judgment, the harshness that gets reflected back to us, and this is the reason we are first going to work to reduce your judgment of other people. By getting out of the habit of critically judging others, you'll be getting out of the habit of being hard on yourself as well.

Still don't understand that we only judge others based on what we judge ourselves on? Think about before you had children. Did you ever look at a baby carrier and think about how good or bad one was? Probably not. Once you had your baby, did you then look at other's strollers and think about how good yours was compared to theirs, or how much you liked theirs better than yours? Yes. We judge things that we judge ourselves on, so this is why it's important that we step out of that detrimental cycle and build up ways to be confident in our own choices.

To be able to clear enough space to pursue your passions while being the primary caregiver for your children, you first need to let go of judgment, because it will let you be more flexible and confident.

The biggest fuel in your fire is going to be the pursuit of your passion, which needs to be something you really *want* to do, not something that you think you *should* be doing. To make that happen, you'll need to be tuned into what it is you *want* out of your life, enjoy the choices you make in your life, and let go of what you think others expect of you. You'll have to let go of the notion that you have to say "yes" to everything to stay involved, because you'll need to say "no" to create space for yourself. You'll have to let go of the guilt you had about wanting a break from your children, because you'll need time away from them to pursue an important goal for yourself. You'll have to trust yourself to make the best decisions at the time you need to make them, stepping away from external expectations and instead, listening confidently to your gut instinct.

Move from Judgment to Observation / Curiosity

One of the best ways to counteract an unhealthy habit, according to Charles Duhigg, is to understand its structure—the cue that spurs it on, the habit you have, and the reward you get from it—and then create a new habit in its place. What if we were to start by observing ourselves each time we caught ourselves being judgmental or critical? We don't want to beat ourselves up for judging—no need to judge the judging. But simply observe, find out what it was that you were judging, what you were thinking, how you were feeling, what that judgment might be saying about what you really want or need, and what your brain is gaining by sticking with that habit. By starting with observation, we will quickly get to the point where we stop the judgment before it turns into outward criticism. I've included an exercise on some common judgment triggers for moms in the workbook that you can get by contacting us at www.flexmombook.com.

Once that becomes a habit and you start to notice your own patterns, replace the observation with a sense of curiosity. Things that you tend to judge are probably things that are different than what you consider normal or right for you. But more often than not, there is a reason someone else is living a different life than the one you chose—they're living the one that is normal and right for them. Be curious about those people or things. The woman who chooses to stay at home even though she has an Ivy League degree—wonder what made her do that, and how she is finding the experience? The woman who wears a power suit and high heels to school drop-off—wonder what it is she does, where she gets her energy? The family who eats free breakfast at school even though they can afford to eat at home (or can they?)—what motivates them to get to school so early, and how does the free breakfast thing work anyway?

Judgment often stems from a gap in understanding, and curiosity is the thing that can help bridge the gap. Even the mommy wars, the ones pitting stay-at-home moms against working moms, come from a disconnect. There is no way to fully appreciate what it's like to be a mom on the opposite side of the parenting model, unless you've been a person who's done them both. Working moms juggle their jobs and their households and, while they don't know what stay-at-home moms do all day, they are busy running their own lives and probably don't make the time to ask a stay-at-home mom what she does. The same goes for stay-at-home moms who do not inherently understand the working mom's juggling act. This disconnect can lead to judgment, so if you're finding yourself judging others, take the time to be curious. Wonder what their life might be like, what makes them need to do certain things—and if you have the time, go ahead and strike up a conversation. In the meantime, support each other in the roles that you have all chosen. And because you have chosen to be the primary caregiver to your children, be confident in your choice, be curious about how to maximize that role, be present in it, and enjoy it!

Lessen the Labels

Labels make it easier to find similarities and order in a world that is, quite frankly, chaotic. It's understandable that, especially when it comes to managing the unpredictability of raising small children, we look to labels to help us make sense of things. However, labels also come with a downside: they lead us to be inflexible and judgmental when we want to blur the lines.

I decided when I was pregnant that I would breastfeed my children. I'd heard all about the benefits of breast milk—the immunity boost, the GI tract being filled with all the necessary probiotics and nutrients—and I knew that my mom managed to do it with all three of her children, so I thought: why not me, too? My first child was able to breastfeed quite easily. Sweet, I thought, I was now a breastfeeding mom and was giving my daughter all these amazing benefits. When I made it to my goal of breastfeeding for a year, my daughter was old enough to transition onto regular milk and I weaned her off the breast. My second child had no problem breastfeeding either, but unfortunately, she developed such bad GI issues that for the first seven months of her life she wouldn't take a supplemental bottle, and then started having such an upset stomach that I had to cut out everything but chicken and rice from my diet to see what was going on with her. My poor baby was crying out in pain around the clock, and by the time I started losing weight from this restricted diet, not to mention losing my mind, I knew I ought to bottle-feed her the super hypoallergenic formula just to make her better. Oh, but the agonizing decision this was! I knew all about the benefits of breastfeeding and I wanted to desperately make it to my self-imposed goal to be a "breastfeeding mom," despite seeing quite clearly that my supply wasn't working out for her. Despite the stress, the lack of sleep, and my daughter's clear discomfort, it took me another week to let go of the notion of "breast is best" and I only changed to formula feeding when my husband sent me physically out of the house overnight, telling me he'd make sure she didn't starve. She did well, and within 24 hours of being on the formula, all of her symptoms subsided. For me, this was a powerful lesson in the importance of recognizing the downside of labels, and being less attached to them. While being a breastfeeding mom was a helpful label to motivate me through the sleepy nights, I needed to see it for what it was (a guide) and needed to be confident and flexible enough to step away from it and quickly listen to my instincts about what was best for my child and me.

Several classic studies of race, intellect, and socio-economics have shown that labels shape perception, and those labels become the dominant lens that we view those people through. Sure, you may judge others and keep them at arm's distance because of some label you've put on them—if you're into helicopter parenting, you may not want your kids to be best buds with free rangers who are alone on the playground several miles away—but you may miss out on opportunities to learn from their stories. The most challenging thing that happens is that, if we regularly label others, we tend to be people who are rigid about the labels we put on ourselves as well. Hand in hand with our tendency to judge, since we now wear this particular label and believe that this one thing is the "right" way to be, is the fact that—when something happens one day to make us suddenly feel we are not living up to those "right" standards—we are much more prone to beat ourselves up and judge ourselves harshly. We are fixed, and become highly inflexible when we live our lives wearing strict labels. What are some of the parenting labels that make you feel good? What about some parenting labels that make you cringe, judge, or back away? Do any images come to mind when you read these labels?

Overachiever	Working Mom	Perfect Kids
Home schooling	SAHM	Church Mom
Fashionable	Yoga Mom	Independent
Soccer Mom	Pinterest Mom	PTA Mom
Room Mom	Artsy	Party Mom
Breastfeeding	Strict	Spiritual
Bottle Feeding	Strong	Co-Sleeping
Free-Range	Tiger Mom	Crafty
Helicopter	Attachment	Babywearing
Blogger Mom	Stage Mom	Mompreneur
Organic	Work at Home	Single Mom
Tech Free	Overprotective	Divorced

Labels are helpful when you consider them a guide, so be conscious of whether you're using them to support you, or whether you're using them to create a judgmental, better-than/worse-than hierarchy in your mind. If you find yourself blurring the edges of a label you like to wear for yourself, be okay with it. Know that you will be happier if you adopt a mindset of non-judgment and flexibility. As you move from being a stay-at-home mom to being a Flex Mom, you too, will have to shed the label of being only one thing—the Flex Mom lives in a flexible world in between two previously strict models for motherhood. Be gentle with yourself as you step into your new multi-dimensional role, and please be gentle with others as they follow their own path.

Know Your Own Strengths and Traits

Once you've prepared yourself to be open-minded about others, and therefore yourself, it's time to begin exploring what it is that you are all about. Instead of using other people's definitions of success and other people's labels, let's take a moment to define who you are, what you enjoy about your life, and what you want to make of your experience.

Why do this? Well, mostly because it's probably been a long time since you reassessed what it is that you are really good at, what it is you need to be the best version of yourself, and what it is that you want out of your life. Once you are confident and know your self, the judgment that comes from outside, the guilt that gnaws at you and makes you feel inadequate, will be gone. You won't worry about the boundaries and labels that others have created before you, and instead you'll be confidently attuned to your own internal compass to navigate the daily decisions you make—especially as your children grow and your family changes.

The reason we begin with strengths is that, no matter what lifestyle you want to create, you will have to rely on certain strengths of yours to uphold that lifestyle. Parents tend to be great about knowing their children's strengths, because they spend so much time observing them and finding ways to motivate them to do their best—or to just get them to do what you want them to. If your child has a love of learning, you would make sure you found new ways to feed into that enthusiasm and wouldn't have them just sit in a corner playing the same easy game over and over again. If your child has a great sense of gratitude, you would thank them for remembering to hang their backpacks up and empty the papers and lunchbox in an effort to speak their language and reinforce positive behavior. There is no reason for us to not be armed with that same information about our own strengths, so we can play into those strengths as we craft the outcomes we desire.

As I transitioned into the Flex Mom lifestyle, I discovered that one of my concerns was that I would get so focused on my goals that I would pull back from nurturing my children; or, even worse, that I wouldn't even be aware I wasn't present for them when they needed me. The upside of uncovering my strengths was that, as it turned out, one of my top five strengths is my capacity to love and be loved, where "the people to whom you feel most close are the same people who feel most close to you." Knowing this gave me the confidence to continue pursuing my goals, because it meant that if I was feeling really close with my children, then they would in all likelihood be feeling close with me. It was great reinforcement for me to regularly check in with my gut instinct about how our family is doing, and listen to my intuition on those days when our family feels off or disconnected—I know to trust myself because if I'm not feeling loved, then my husband and/or children probably aren't either, and I can immediately do something to counteract that. Knowing my strengths has been a great tool for me to uphold the close-knit relationships that I want to maintain for myself and for my family, while continuing to pursue my goals.

Of course, you can always guess at your strengths, but one of the easiest ways to figure them out is to spend 15 minutes online checking out the VIA Strengths Survey from the Institute of Character. Once you have these defined, play around a little bit with those listed in your top five—use one strength every day for a week in a new way, for example, or figure out when you use each strength most naturally in your day-to-day life. You want to use your strengths by playing them up, relying on them, building up the "strength muscles" even stronger so you feel confident in what you are good at. Don't spend too much time worrying about your weaknesses, because you can manage these fairly easily—think instead about the way you can use each strength to support your values.

The second key to defining your core self is to understand your inherent personality traits. These are the things that, no matter what your strengths and lifestyle, are inherently programmed and you probably cannot change. You want to understand what these traits are so you can appreciate what you are wired to need, how you are wired to think, and how to treat yourself well within that structure. Knowing your personality traits earlier in the Flex Mom process can help you build the support you need to create the space to pursue your passion—or even just to hit your basic stride. For me, it turns out that I am an introvert. When I was home with a baby and preschooler with a husband who traveled regularly, I felt like it was only natural for a stay-at-home mom to power through on her own, so I took the children with me everywhere. I couldn't understand why I was constantly drained, on a different level than just sleep deprivation, but it all made sense to me when I took the Myers Briggs personality test. Despite being an introvert, I'm very social and I play the role of the family extrovert but, per the definition of introversion, I need time alone to recharge. With two small children with me constantly, I was getting zero time to power myself back up! As soon as we got these results, my husband and I agreed that it made sense to find a way to give me some more alone time. I hired a babysitter to come in once a week so I could have time to run errands by myself, and asked my fellow stay-at-home mom friends to do kid swaps, so I could connect with people for lunch, go to the library and read in silence, take a hike, or do whatever I wanted to do to recharge my batteries all by myself. The support helped me feel much more energetic while my children were little, and allowed me to be a better, more playful parent. It also made me realize how much space I would need to hold for myself to not just feel a basic level of recharge, but to have the mental resources to pursue the goals I had set for myself. It's one of the biggest reasons I waited until both my children were old enough to be in school full time to take on a bigger project like this book, so I could have these child-free days to pursue my goals—while still having enough space in my life to recharge my batteries.

The official Myers Briggs test requires seeing a practitioner to help you decipher your core personality traits, so if that's within your budget and timeframe, I'd highly recommend finding someone near you. There are also plenty of other tools online to discover these traits; while you can do some searches yourself, I've listed some of the best resources I have found thus far at the back of the book. Feel free to check them out.

Define Your Family Values

Values are the things that are central to who you are, who you want to be, and help define the way you live. Making the time to sit down with your partner and discuss family values is an important step in building up the Flex Mom model. By knowing what you stand for as a family, you'll be able to make better decisions about where you want to go with your own passion, as well as which boundaries you're willing to push and which are non-negotiables. As a bonus, once family values are articulated with your children, they can lean on those same values when faced with decisions in their own lives.

There doesn't have to be pressure to separate out each of your values as individuals, because they will get bundled up into the family values—and you can, in one swoop, uphold the ideals that are important to both you and your partner. For example, one of my personal values is a sense of comfort. Looking back at my own upbringing, I am so happy that my mom still lives in the same house I was born and raised in. I love that I have a physical place in this world I can return to, even as an adult, and feel the same comfort and familiarity that I grew up with. For our family, with a husband/father who travels for a living, it was going to be difficult to create that sense of comfort and consistency for our children if we were both working. We made the choice for me to become the primary caregiver for our children so I could spend time shaping our day-to-day, to be a consistent presence in our children's lives, and to give them the same comfort and consistency that I had. There was no need for me to be adamant that my value of comfort was going to have to be part of our family values—it just is part of our family values, because I am one of the two creators of our family.

The reason family values are so helpful to articulate becomes clear in rougher times. It's fine to carry on doing what you're doing without knowing what you stand for, but when something comes up that feels wrong or edgy or challenging, it will be much easier to identify what is going on and correct your course if your values have been articulated. For example, I have never been a particularly good cook. Back when I was growing up, my mother was greatly concerned about my future because I never spent time with her in the kitchen learning how to whip up her amazing Japanese meals, and she thought for sure I'd never survive, let alone be able to raise a family. Fast forward years later, and amazingly, my mother-in-law commented—in a kind way—about just how "domestic" I'd gotten once I had children. I learned how to go beyond boiling a pot of water and throwing a piece of bread in a toaster, and could actually put together a delicious meal and even host a well plated Thanksgiving dinner. While cooking is still not my favorite thing to do, we have multiple family members with food sensitivities and my husband and I decided that it was going to be very important (and much more financially sound) for us to cook at home instead of eating out at specialized restaurants. My husband is a fantastic cook, and we decided to seize the opportunity of home-cooking most of our meals to teach our children where food comes from, the difference between fresh and processed food, and how food goes from farm to table. We tend to cook from conscious sources—including our own backyard garden—and the spark this decision has provided for us has been rewarding. Being aware that home cooking is our family value helps my mindset immensely not just on weekends, when I feel myself resistant to making many meals for many mouths over and over again, but also when I'm busy working on my own projects, pursuing my goals, and would prefer to ignore our need to eat. I take a moment to remember that cooking is something we make time for in my home, and because this is a lifestyle value that our family chose, I feel less like an underappreciated short order cook, and more like an empowered woman who manages to write a book while still putting home cooked meals on the table for her family.

Sitting down with your partner to articulate the values that drew you together in the first place is a great way to start defining your own family values, those that you want to pass along to your children and those you want to have set the tone for the major decisions each of you make. You can consider asking yourselves what it is you do even though you don't necessarily want to (e.g. cooking, above), what phrases you find yourselves using when chatting with your children, or what it is you find yourselves doing most naturally together. Our family realized we valued persistence when we caught ourselves regularly cheering on the kids, saying, "This family never gives up!" We also realized that one of the biggest ways we show love is to hug and kiss and tell each other how much we love each other, so "we hug often" became another family value. Inspired by Bruce Feiler, we took our list of values and put them on a big board in our living room. In our case, we happened to find one at Target that said pretty much everything we wanted it to say; I'm sure it's possible to have them typed up on a customized online site somewhere to order and hang up. It's amazing when our little ones quote some of our values back to us, like when we try to rush them off to bed and they slow us down, reminding us that we told them in the morning that they could have one dessert today, and "in our family we never break promises, do we?" Where before, I wondered if what I was saying as a parent today was consistent with what I said as a parent yesterday, having outlined these values now keeps me and my family in consistent alignment with what we stand for—even when, and especially when, things get busier as I pursue my goals.

If you're not sure where to start defining your values, you can access the values worksheet in the workbook I've created. In the workbook be some questions you can answer together to start the process; there will also be a list of sample values for you to look through. Picking from a list isn't always the best way to finalize the values process, as you really want to listen to your intuition about what fits you best, but it's a great place to start. You can do what's called a "values ladder" where you pick a bunch of values that resonate the most with you, and, starting at the bottom, compare each word to the one above it. If you were in a pickle and had to make a decision based on one value over the other, which would you choose? The one you'd value more continues to move up the ladder, until you eventually have a list of your values in priority order, with the rough aim of having a list of maybe 8–12 of your most important values. After you spend some time on this exercise, put the list away for a few days and see if anything else jumps out at you that you want to add, and then make a decision about how you want to share those values with your family unit so you can all be on the same page.

To step into the mindset of the Flex Mom and be able to clear enough space to pursue your passions while being the primary caregiver for your children, you want to change your tendency to judge. The Flex Mom's goals will be something you really *want* to do, not something that you think you *should* be doing, so it's important to shed any guilt you have about not living up to external expectations and learn to trust your own internal compass instead. By adopting habits of observation and curiosity about other's values and expectations, by learning about and defining your strengths, personality traits, and family values, you'll be able to better differentiate what's yours and what's not yours. Soon, you'll have the confidence to make decisions that support what you need and do best, and this confidence is the first step in the framework to build up a Flex Mom.

CHAPTER 4
LOVE YOURSELF

"To keep the body in good health is a duty... otherwise we shall not be able to keep our mind strong and clear."
—Buddha

M y husband is an airline pilot, so we've traveled quite a lot, and are used to the safety advice that flight attendants recite before takeoff. But if you really, really listen to their message, you'll realize that we ought to heed their directions: in case of an emergency, we are to secure our own oxygen masks first before helping children put theirs on. As it happens, in real life, it is imperative that we take care of ourselves first, because we are better parents to our children when we are healthy and happy.

I don't mean you should deprioritize your children entirely and ignore them in dire circumstances, you understand. But I do mean that you can take a shower once a day, you can find time to exercise, you can eat real meals, you can take a moment to have an adult conversation. You can't do everything, but you can do almost anything you want to, on most days anyway. That is why, in the last chapter, you started exploring the values that you and your family stand for, so you know what you, as a family, feel is most important to you, and so you can spend less time worrying about things you don't actually care about.

In this chapter, you'll start prioritizing your body. Your body is the vehicle that carries your amazing brain and the passions that you have inside you. The habits you build to take care of your body are similar to the habits you will need to keep focused on pursuing your Flex Mom goals—especially if things get challenging. Plus, by boosting your body's levels of well-being, you'll be maximizing your happiness and, therefore, chances of success. Researcher and positive psychology expert Shawn Achor has shown that happiness is a precursor to success, and if we want to be successful caregivers for our children while also pursuing our own goals, we cannot ignore our happiness. It turns out that about 50% of our happiness comes from a biologically predetermined level. Sure, circumstances and intentional "happiness boosting" activities also affect our happiness, but our bodies, our biology, dictate the largest portion of our happiness. That is why the next step in the Flex Mom process is making sure that we build habits to let us meet our basic human needs to sleep, eat, and move well. I'll add sauciness to that, as I know there are way too many not-really-jokes about married couples with children letting their sex life disappear. These habits are another layer in the foundation of your Flex Mom life, because you want to make sure your body and mind stay healthy and happy as you continue to pursue your goals. You don't want to find that you are so engrossed in pursuing your goal that you forget to take care of your body, and then get sick or start dragging—that will absolutely get in the way of your forward momentum.

How do you start building habits that lead you to take better care of your body? I like to use one of the seven principles in Shawn's book *The Happiness Advantage*, regarding happiness at work, and apply that principle to managing your life and your home. It's called the Zorro Circle, and is all about limiting your focus to small, manageable goals that can then expand your sense of control. And if anything is a huge mascot for a lack of control, it would be children and child rearing—children who can easily derail any progress you want to make towards your big goals. Much like Zorro started his training by defending one small circle around himself, train yourselves to tackle the small, manageable goals in front of you, which will lead to taking better care of your bodies, which then will lead you to higher levels of happiness, which will support the successful pursuit of your Flex Mom goals.

My goal in this chapter is to help you make concrete changes in your life. You all know intellectually that it's good to get 8 hours of sleep, you know vegetables are better for you than a pint of ice cream, and you know that you're supposed to exercise. But unfortunately, just because you *know* you ought to be doing these things doesn't mean that you're *actually* doing them. It takes about three weeks to build a habit, so define the changes you want to focus on for the duration of that time and use this idea of little victories, keeping Zorro's battle circles under your own control, until you establish these as habits—if they are important to you.

Sleep is Critical to Your Well Being

I remember when my daughter was a newborn. I was overly cautious and, in addition to waking up when she needed to be fed, I'd often wake myself up in a fright and check on her through the night to make sure she was still breathing. I got so tired that one time, just after she transitioned from a pack and play in my bedroom to her own big girl crib, I woke up, picked her up, and walked with her back into her bedroom—but as I pushed open her door, I found her already in the crib. I'd completely hallucinated that I was carrying my baby.

Especially after having spent the first years of each of my children's lives being a zombie, I am very proud to declare that I love sleep. I used to make fun of my parents for going to bed at 9pm as we were growing up; I thought they were utterly uncool, and that staying up past midnight was the thing to do. Now, I cherish the nights I get the kids to bed, have some alone time, and can crawl into bed with a book by 9pm. This is not about getting old—I'll reframe that thought and just call this wisdom.

Science has proven that sleep is not just something we do when we are too weak to carry on. Sleep is your body's opportunity to heal itself physically and emotionally. While you are sleeping, your body heals its own heart and blood vessels, it regulates the balance of hormones that manage your hunger levels and insulin levels, it releases hormones that manage your growth and works on muscle and brain repair, and your immune system also relies on sleep to help keep you healthy. And as any parent who has experienced the lack of sleep accompanying the first few months of a child's life knows, sleep also helps your brain make decisions more quickly, helps you pay attention, be creative, and basically avoid the brain fog and depression that can come with too little sleep. Brain fog and depression aren't the best ways to start pursuing your own passion or setting your own goals, because you probably won't be in tune with your gut instinct and have the gumption to hold space for yourself. This is why the Flex Mom begins taking care of her body by creating healthy sleep patterns.

I tell my children that if I have to wake them up in the morning for school, it's a sign that their bodies actually want more sleep, which means they're not getting enough and need to get to bed earlier. So for us to do this as adults, think about the last time that you woke up on your own, without an alarm clock, and without a kid poking you on the forehead asking for breakfast. If you don't have a memory of such a time, that means it's time to set up a new sleep routine that lets your body get the rest it needs, so you can be mentally sharp enough and in tune with your instincts to continue making the choices you need as a Flex Mom. Plus, we will be talking in a later chapter about setting boundaries to clear space for you to pursue your goals, and guarding your sleep is one of the easiest ways to begin learning how to set boundaries. So try this: give yourself a bedtime. After suggesting this idea, I went online to make sure it wasn't a horrible suggestion— and it turns out Dr. Mehmet Oz lists not having an adult bedtime as his Deadly Habit 7! So go ahead and set a bedtime, for real. No, you don't have to yell at yourself for not sticking with it like you would your child, but give yourself one.

To start, let's go with the average recommended 8 hours of sleep and work backwards. What time do you need to wake up in the morning to start your routine without feeling like you're rushing through a shower, breakfast, and coffee? Say in your ideal world you like to wake up, stretch, make a cup of coffee without kids around so you don't have to find it lukewarm in the microwave hours later, and then are better prepared to handle your kids with a smile. Does that mean that 6am wakeups would work? Whatever time works for you, write that morning time down. Then count back 8 hours (or however much sleep your body needs to get to feel rested) and write that down as your lights-off bedtime.

Track back another 30 minutes from that, and use that as your "bedtime routine" time, with no more cell phones or technology. This is an important point to remember, because the blue light of electronic devices suppresses the normal release of melatonin that happens at night, and this dip in melatonin will keep you awake longer, cutting into your quality sleep time. As part of your healthy sleep routine, plan to be brushing your teeth and washing your face and getting into jammies about 30 minutes before your bedtime. Do some deep breathing or gratitude exercises to get your brain thinking about relaxing. If you enjoy reading, pick up a real book or magazine, or even an e-reader that does not emit blue light. Stick with this bedtime routine for several weeks to let your body get used to the sleep, and see if you notice a difference. The idea is that if you can establish healthy, regular bedtime habits, you should be able to open your eyes in the morning with more of a smile and less of a scowl as the obnoxious alarm clock blares.

For example, say you want to be awake by 7am.

You would head to bed at 10pm, with no more technology.

You would turn the lights off at 10:30pm. It can take 20–30 minutes for most people to fall asleep, so you would probably be asleep by 11pm.

You would wake up by 7am, refreshed.

In the back of this book are several resources if you'd like to learn more about sleep. There will also be a number of people reading this who, despite their best efforts, have challenges with sleep. Don't let these go unchecked for too long—please consult a physician for some advice on what might be happening. Your thyroid and adrenals might be out of whack (technical term, I know), your body may need extra melatonin support, you may not have enough iron stores in your body, causing restless legs, your brain might be processing so much subconsciously that you need to do extra training to relax. You may still have small children who wake up at night; there are ways to encourage them to get the rest they need, so you get your sleep as well. If your children are still napping and you need some extra rest, let go of your to-do list and prioritize your health by napping with them. Sleep is a crucial part of taking care of your body, and you want to have your body operating at high capacity in order to create the lifestyle you want to have.

Eating Will Affect Your Mood

After my second child was born, I went through another 16 months of very little sleep. My baby had a sensitive system, and I just assumed that it was because of this lack of sleep that I was operating in a brain fog. That misbelief continued until my older daughter's sensitive system came into focus and we started eliminating certain foods from her diet. (Apparently John and I breed gastrointestinally sensitive children.) Out of solidarity—because what four-year-old wants to be the one person in the family who has to eat something different?—I went off gluten with her. And within a week, my brain fog started lifting.

I had no idea that the dairy and gluten sensitivities that my children were exhibiting came from none other than me! I had no food sensitivities before the children were born, and had only heard anecdotally of moms gaining them during pregnancy, so I never considered it as an option for me. But, like many other parts of parenting, here was another surprise. The triggers for the transition were probably the pregnancies, and the stress that they had on my body, but I don't really know what caused it. What I do know is that being aware of my food sensitivities, and being more mindful about the foods I was putting into my body, made a tremendous difference in my ability to function through the day. This led to us being a lot more proactive about cooking our own meals. The gluten-free movement kicked off in earnest at about the same time that we removed it from our diet, so it became easier to find alternative foods at grocery stores and find suitable foods at restaurants—but it's expensive! So we started making a lot more of our food at home, and had to figure out how to fit that routine into our daily lives. Much as cooking isn't my favorite thing to do, it was important to us that we not cloud our brains or cause GI distress by eating foods that we were sensitive to. Our family declared that home cooking was going to be an important value for us, so now I make sure that even while I'm pursuing my own goals, I make time to cook meals for the family and nourish us in a way that keeps our bodies and brains functioning well.

This shouldn't surprise many of you—feeding your children is a basic part of any parent's life. The Flex Mom is the person who prioritizes child care, so will often be the one who is responsible for putting the food on the plate, and while this is a generalization, she is probably going to be doing more home cooking than dining out. This means that, even while you are pursuing your goals, you will have to feed your family regular meals to support their growth. It makes it much easier to come up with systems around food to take the stress out of it—having systems reduces the time and mental space you use thinking about what to cook and how to make time to cook it, leaving you more capacity for your goals. What's working for you right now in your meal planning and prep? What is not working?

My friend Liz ran around so much with the kids after school that she'd often still be out when her husband got home from work. Yet, even though he got home first, he didn't know what was for dinner, so he wouldn't start prepping anything. That frustrated her so much that she decided to take a big picture frame, insert a colorful piece of paper and use dry erase markers to write out their weekly meal plan. They would then use Instacart, a grocery delivery service, over the weekend and order all the foods needed to make those meals through the week. Now, if her husband gets home before her, he's already starting to get the meals ready and the evening goes much more smoothly. Wins for everyone.

Another friend, Grace, talked with her family and decided that they wanted to cook most of their meals, but she was exhausted from breastfeeding their youngest child through the night and chasing after the toddler, while still managing to drive the older child to and from school and classes. Since her husband doesn't enjoy cooking at all, they decided that they would designate Sunday mornings as Daddy-kids time, and she would get the house to herself for several hours, blasting her favorite music and dancing around the kitchen while she batch-cooked meals. They capitalized on Black Friday sales and bought a deep-freeze to fit in their garage, and they now store meals for later in the week in that freezer for easy defrosting.

Yet another friend, Suzanne, has designated days of the week for certain meal types. She has "Daddy's Special Sundays" and "Pasta Mondays" and "Taco Tuesdays" so within that broad structure, she finds a new (or tried and true favorite) recipe to fit the theme for each day of the week. Like Liz, Suzanne also writes the meal plan down on a weekly calendar, so everyone in the family knows what to expect from the week ahead.

How else can you make healthier eating a defensible habit? If the idea of chemical-filled foods grosses you out, download a list of "the dirty dozen" and make sure you buy organic versions of those items. If, in theory, you want to serve more fish but the kids aren't digging it, look into Omega-3 supplements for the family. If you don't typically like letting the kids watch TV but decide that feeding them home cooked meals is more important, be flexible, make it easy on yourself, and turn on the TV for 30 minutes to distract them while you cook. If you are the main chef of the family but need a break from the kitchen once in a while to motivate yourself, create a calendar and get over the guilt of "unhealthy foods" and make every Friday a pizza night. Sit down and figure out just how much you want to cook, decide what your rotating roster of regular meals you enjoy cooking are, assign meals for the week, get the shopping done in bulk, and most importantly, figure out what's getting in the way of accomplishing those things—and tackle those items so you can make this a new habit for you and your family.

Make Time to Shake That Booty

Just the other night, I was at book club and one of the moms lamented about how difficult it was to find time to exercise. We ended up talking about each of our methods, and it turns out that if it's important to us, we get it done. One girlfriend knows she gets in a serious mental funk without exercise, so ends up pushing 100lbs of double stroller plus a huge dog on her daily morning runs just to get it in; on the days her husband is home to help out, she goes on longer, faster runs by herself.

Are you that person who needs defined exercise, and wants to find time? If you're a social person, call a friend once a week and take your kids on a run, let them ride bikes while you jog alongside, walk together with your kids in strollers—or even join a local Stroller Strides group. If you are motivated by classes, look around at the local community centers or gyms (particularly those with daycares for your little ones!) and sign yourself up for several classes per week. You can explain to your children that Mommy wants to stay strong and healthy so she has more energy to play with them. If you enjoy time to yourself, consider getting a DVD (am I dating myself? Maybe these are all streaming videos now) that you can pop onto the TV, or invest in a machine that you can put in a corner of your house. If you're an early morning riser and your partner can watch the children, set the alarm a bit earlier and knock out the exercise so you feel great through the day.

No matter what, on the days that you commit time into your calendar to exercise, wake up in the morning and put on your workout outfit to limit the excuses you have for not getting your body moving. Shawn Achor calls this his "20 second rule," where you lower the barrier to doing what you want to do, making it very likely that you will go ahead and do it. Even if it only takes you an extra 20 seconds to grab your exercise gear in the morning instead of putting on your regular clothes, that barrier may be enough to stop you from getting out the door to get your body moving. So, make it as easy as possible for yourself by setting up exactly what it is you want to do through the week, making a commitment with a friend to show up, and laying out what you're going to wear on those days ahead of time. You want to exercise, so you simply go ahead and do it. These same habits—of setting up a schedule, making a commitment, and lowering your barrier to starting—are going to be helpful when you decide on your goals and start to pursue them. You will be operating within time constraints and aiming to be highly efficient because you still want to prioritize your time with your children, so you'll be working during the limited times when your children are otherwise occupied. You want to make the most of the time you have, so you will benefit by making your actions efficient and intentional. While writing this book, I made sure that my laptop and stack of reference books and notebooks were sitting in a pile right by my workstation, so that, on my designated writing days, I had no excuse to search for this or that item to delay when I needed to get started.

Another woman at book club, a stay-at-home mom, didn't care so much about explicit exercise and didn't want to join a gym or a class, so she decided to lead a more active lifestyle by taking the stairs and parking her car further away from the store, and that worked for her to maintain a feeling of healthy activity. Which, actually, makes some sense. Our attitude towards what qualifies as exercise matters, so while cardio and strength training exercises are important, if you're aware of how much you're moving, there's no need to beat yourself up that you yet again didn't make it to the gym because your kid was sick. A cool study by Crum and Langer tracked 84 female room attendants at a hotel and found that even though the behavior of these women did not change (they cleaned rooms), the ones who were told that the work that they did met the recommended definition of an active lifestyle actually had lower weight, lower blood pressure, body fat, and BMI after only four weeks! Four weeks after they were simply made aware that they were in fact living an active lifestyle, with no other changes!

This can offer some reassurance for stay-at-home moms and Flex Moms alike. FitBits and movement trackers are all the rage right now, tallying many of our statistics. Having received one as a gift, I was pleasantly surprised to find just how many steps I took during the course of an average day taking care of the house—I easily achieved the recommended 10,000 steps between picking up toys, chasing after children, walking them to and from school, wearing a path between my refrigerator and the sink to make a billion meals and snacks in a day. These steps aren't a full substitute for the mental and physical boost I get when I make it to the cardio class or the yoga studio, but for my daily routine, it certainly was reassuring to know that I moved a lot more than I thought I did—and made me aware that when I do sit more (like I'm doing to write this book), I need to plan for more time to make it to an exercise class or take a walk. Again, getting into the habit of exercise is something I am encouraging you to do now before you add a new goal to your life, because it will be very tempting to toss everything aside when you're excited about pursuing your goals—when in fact, continuing to exercise *as* you pursue your goals is one of the very things that will continue to energize you and keep you healthy, both mentally and physically.

How are you getting your body moving, and what is standing in the way of getting it done so you feel stronger? What change can you make in your daily life for the next few weeks to establish a new habit around the exercise that you want to do?

It's Okay for Moms to be Feminine Beings

Once we become mothers, it's very easy to forget, through all the exhaustion and chaos of parenting, about the sex and sexuality that actually got us to be mothers in the first place. A woman named Amy mentioned to me that her husband had cooked her a fancy meal on a Saturday night, complete with an expensive bottle of wine; when she told her mom friends about it, their reaction was "oooooooh, he wanted to get some!"—as if she wouldn't want to have sex with her husband herself. Yet when we were single, or even pre-kids, we never would have joked with friends about not wanting to have sex. One of the biggest draws that we had toward our partner was probably the sexual chemistry.

I had a great conversation about this issue of sex and femininity with Jaime Myers, owner of Shine Life Design and a coach who taught for PAX Programs across the US for 11 years. We talked about the three powerful feminine models of empress, siren, and mother, and realized that it's the siren and empress that we often forget about when we are heavily in mother mode—when we are busy caring for and looking out for others, when it's very easy to sacrifice our sense of self. Keep in mind that being a mother is still a very powerful model, one that lets you ask your spouse "Hey, I'm grabbing my jacket, want me to get yours?" which is definitely positive and well-rounded. It is very distinct from when we tip into mother-ing mode, a controlling mode where you demand that they "put on another layer because it's cold outside!" which is off-putting to everyone on the receiving end—especially when we do that to our partners, unaware.

Still, it's easy to forget about treating ourselves well as women unless we shift our attention back to the other models of powerful femininity. What makes you feel a bit more glamorous and in touch with your beautiful, confident, or playful self? These shouldn't be things like "when I weigh 25 pounds less" or "only when I wear a bikini"—things that are not easy or realistic to do regularly. One friend, Page, says that she feels most beautiful when her hair looks good, and feels sexy when she wears something that outlines her hips. She now takes a little extra time each morning to make sure her hair looks the way she wants; when she goes on a rare date with her man, she makes sure to wear the outfits that trace her curves, because as soon as her man touches them, it's confirmation of her feeling of sexiness. For a different friend, Danna, she realized a great pair of underwear makes her feel feminine and sexy, as does a heartfelt compliment from her husband when he sees her wearing them. You bet she invests in good underwear and treats it well so she doesn't have to settle for cotton briefs any more. For me, I love the feeling of looking down at my toes when they have a fresh pedicure—so I get fairly regular pedicures, often gel ones because they last longer and don't chip—and that comes straight from the family maintenance budget and not the luxury line item. These little things you do to treat yourself better, like swiping a touch of lip gloss on your lips before you head to the playground, or wearing a sexier nightie to bed, are physical reminders to maintain the mental attitude of femininity. We are emerging from that second wave of feminism, which proposed that strong and powerful women should compete in the workforce with men, and the Flex Mom no longer has to compete with men to be powerful at work. The Flex Mom is busy being powerful as a woman, as she prioritizes her children and pursues her own dreams. What is the thing, the small habit, that you can do most regularly to remind you of your feminine power, to keep you feeling saucy and confident and playful, and feeling like you don't have to push push push through the daily grind to compete anymore?

(Side note: If you are someone who believes that femininity is weak, think again. Look at models like Danielle LaPorte, Marie Forleo, Elizabeth Gilbert, Brené Brown, and Michelle Obama. These women maintain their grace, femininity, and simply ooze strength and influence. And you can bet they all make time for sleep, exercise, and eating well.)

In this chapter, we talked about establishing small changes that can be defended over and over again until they become habits, in the realm of sleep, eating, moving, and femininity. When we prioritize self-care, we are in a better position to be happier people and parents, and have more mental and physical capacity to stick up for the values and lifestyle that are important to us. In addition to those benefits, the habits you build in practicing self-care are some of the same habits that you will use to create and maintain the space you need to pursue your goals. These healthy habits are the building blocks upon which you build the next layer of the Flex Mom process, of defining your passion and setting bigger goals for yourself outside of your home.

CHAPTER 5
EXPRESS YOUR GOALS

"Setting goals is the first step in turning the invisible into the visible."

—Tony Robbins

Remember when you used to have a career? You got up in the morning to the sound of your alarm clock, you brushed your teeth and washed your face, you ate breakfast and got dressed in work clothes—you prepared to tackle the day and move towards the goals that you set for the day. Maybe today was the day you had to hit a certain sales target. Maybe you had to prepare statements or deliver a speech, or maybe you had a full day ahead of you caring for patients. You had to meet hard and fast deadlines, and had people expecting you to do great things—people who held you accountable and who you did not want to disappoint.

Do you remember the energy you used to have to drive towards those goals? You may have been tired, may have needed an extra cup of coffee some mornings, but you had motivation, energy, movement to get through those days because these little achievements and little goals were steps towards an even bigger goal. A "good job" from your colleague or recognition from your bosses seemed like building blocks towards the ultimate promotion or raise you wanted, another notch in the fabulous reputation that you built for yourself. You needed to put your best professional foot forward every day, and you'd have a sense of satisfaction that you achieved something, that you were accomplishing the goals that you'd put your mind to. You were like a horse in a race: blinders on, focused on a goal.

Now imagine that same energy, stuck on a hamster wheel. Running full tilt to stand still.

That's you, parenting.

The same thing, day after day. Breakfast cooked, dishes need to be cleaned up. Snack made, crumbs need to be cleared. Lunch time rolls around, same thing. Oh, and how about dinner when your significant other joins you? Yep, let's make another healthy delicious meal, just with a bit more pressure because the can of tuna you want to shovel into your mouth instead of cooking again simply won't cut it. Kid eats, kid spills, kid clothes need to be washed, dried, folded, and put away. Kid poops, kid needs to get wiped. All. Day. Every. Single. Day. It's absolutely mind numbing.

It's even worse when that's all you have to your days. I don't want to make it sound like stay-at-home parents live in misery; we absolutely are lucky that we get to spend so much time with our children and experience many moments of total bliss and adoration for the little beings in our lives. In fact, for some people, it absolutely is a calling to be a mother, and they parent effortlessly and joyfully. They may be bleary eyed when their young one comes crawling into their bed at 2am, but they take them in with open arms and enjoy the cuddles. They dress their children in nice clothing and take care to do their hair just so, and don't mind when clothing gets dirty. They don't go crazy when their children don't know how to spell their last name perfectly by age five, but make it a game to teach them eventually, and the children know it's just good fun. In essence, it truly is their calling and they derive pleasure and purpose out of raising their children single-mindedly, and it is a miracle to behold. I have nothing but admiration for parents like this; I am not one of them and I wish I could have been. It seems like a much more joyful and fun way to be! It's just that for me, and for quite a number of other parents, it's simply difficult to give so much of myself, in such a repetitive way, to a small child without any larger sense of purpose outside of my home.

Still, even for these effortless parents, there is value in this part of the Flex Mom process: setting goals that support your sense of self. When I was recently at a baby shower, I met a charismatic brunette named Addison, whose kindness drew me to sit next to her. During the course of conversation, topics at the table shifted to motherhood and child rearing, and the difficulties of being stay-at-home moms or working moms. It turned out Addison's mother was one of these effortless parents, who made her children her everything, and Addison greatly appreciated the warm memories of her nurturing stay-at-home mother. Then, she sat up straight and said, "But I decided ages ago that I could never be a full time stay-at-home mom—once my youngest brother left for college, my mom fell into a super long depression." Addison's mother confided in her that she had focused for so long on raising her children that she didn't know who she was anymore. She ended up spending about 15 years in a funk, effectively waiting for her first grandchildren to be born—and now that they live close by, her mother got a renewed sense of purpose and has emerged from depression. It was great for her to see her mother feel so much better, but those lengthy sad years are what Addison never wanted to experience, and until we spoke, she hadn't even considered the idea of the Flex Mom way of structuring her life. Instead, she had been struggling through the daily conflict of wanting to spend more time with her kids while working hard at her career –primarily to maintain her own identity.

It seems that for stay-at-home parents, and even for effortless stay-at-home parents, there is benefit in shifting your definition of success away from the pre-children definition to something more personal, and then actively choosing what it is you want to do for yourselves.

Accepting the Hamster Wheel

I wrote in a holiday card the year my eldest child was born that my view of success had changed—that I went from leading a life full of emails, phone calls, projects, and worldly accomplishments to realizing that if I shower, eat three meals, and have the kitchen cleaned before bed I've had a rock star day. What about you? What were your prior expectations of yourself, when you were a professional? And now that you have been a parent for a while, what are your non-negotiables that, if you meet them, make you feel like you've had a great day? I know that my new definition of success worked for me because it allowed me to disconnect from my prior ideals—ideals that made me grumpy because they made me feel like my kids were taking away my ability to email my friends back immediately or have uninterrupted phone calls, things I thought were important when I was not yet a parent. Now I know my basic desires as a parent/human—to feel clean, to feel like I was worth the time it took to make some food (plus it usually meant I socialized over at least one of those meals), and to be able to wake up and peacefully make a cup of coffee to start my morning. It cleared the space I needed to focus on being with my children, to learn how their brains worked and see what they liked to eat and how they liked to play. Meeting my basic definition of success let me be in a much better state of flow with my kids, as they became my new project, my new curiosity—I felt more like the effortless parent, and like maybe it *was* my calling to be their mother.

After making peace with my "new definition of success" and then going through another pregnancy and subsequent newborn-survival-year, I went through a rougher period of time that led me to a breakthrough. I found myself fraying at the edges, wholly unsatisfied with what had previously worked to keep me satisfied: taking a shower and eating like a normal person and having a clean kitchen by the end of the day. My children were wonderful—if awful sleepers for their young lives—and stimulating and vivacious and lovely and all that you'd want your children to be. I'd shifted my diet and gotten out of the brain fog that was brought on by food sensitivities. I was running a women's social group on the side, one that was akin to the stuff I loved doing when life coaching. Still, I wasn't as happy as I knew I could be. Eventually I admitted to my husband that this stay-at-home parenting thing was mentally tough for me, but given our family values and my husband's travel schedule, going back to work wasn't really an option either—nor did I think I had it in me to do a job just to escape my children, especially when I knew that they'd be in school full time in just a few years. I kind of felt yucky. I had chosen this path of stay-at-home parenting and wasn't ready to admit defeat, but the longer I stuck with it, the more trapped on the hamster wheel I felt.

That's when I realized that there was no point in fighting the hamster wheel. Repetition is a necessary part of parenting, of simply having a household, and it certainly is a very normal part of children's developmental stages. I wanted a household, and I wanted to help my kids develop. Instead of fighting the inevitable and getting frustrated, I should simply find a way to manage the repetition, accept that the hamster wheel is only one part of life, and remember that I can find my meaning on a different track. It is this parallel track that Flex Moms need to create and pursue to feel fulfilled—and that parallel track doesn't necessarily have to be a career (though it could be).

The Parallel Track to Your Hamster Wheel

The crux of the Flex Mom is this division of the tracks. You spin the hamster wheel, and you also develop a parallel track that opens your field of view beyond the circular track to allow you to run freely towards a goal—a goal that fuels your passions and fits within the lifestyle you want to live. The energy you get from running on the parallel track will help you spin your hamster wheel. The Flex Mom flows between raising children and being lit up with excitement about the other stuff she has going on.

The goals a Flex Mom sets should be a stretch but also realistic to achieve given your actual time and support. They are things you will probably be good at doing. Most importantly, they should reflect something that you really *want* to do—not something that you think you *should* be doing. This is a goal for you, something that lights your fire.

I was lucky to have a community of friends and coaches who I could bounce ideas around with, to reflect back to me what they were hearing and help me see myself more clearly, much more quickly than I would have had I done this alone. When you identify and begin pursuing goals that are in alignment with your passion, the rest of the things you feel are missing will follow—your sense of self, your hobbies, and your connections—in particular because you will learn skills later in this process that will hold the space for you and support you.

The rewarding thing about setting a goal is that it doesn't mean that you are putting off your happiness until you actually achieve that goal; goals are a means towards happiness. As happiness researcher Tal Ben-Shahar says in his book *Happier*, it's not the attaining of our goals that makes us happy, but the process of working towards achieving something that is meaningful to us. As he eloquently says, "A goal enables us to experience a sense of being while doing" *(Happier,* p. 71*).*

Different Types of Goals: Feeling, Humble, Big Mamas
Let's first make sure we're talking about the same thing when we talk about goals. In my time working and living in this field of wellness, I've come across different layers of goals which, when selected accurately, tend to build on each other to help you achieve ever bigger goals in your life.

"Feeling" goals are those that help you decide how you want to feel when you're pursuing your "big mama" goals. Imagine yourself when you are your best, as you'd want to be right now. What are you wearing, what are you doing, how are you communicating? Then, start to figure out how it is you feel while you are being that best version of yourself. The reason we do this is that, once you identify those feelings, you can use them as the main criteria for your decision-making process.

This exercise may seem simple at first, but it takes a few steps to get to the real feelings you want to have. For example, say you imagined yourself surrounded by a supportive, close-knit community of adults and children. You might start with a general feeling goal like "love"— but this isn't specific enough. Keep breaking your feeling goals down into the essence of the feeling. So, ask yourself, "How does love make me feel?" You might answer, "safe" or "connected" or "joyful." Maybe those are your feeling goals, or maybe you break those words down another level until you get deep enough to access the feelings you really want to have.

Say you do this process, and you decide that your feeling goals for this year are grace, depth, and joy. You would make choices that support the presence of those feelings in your life. For grace, you might make the choice to speak less gossip and prioritize observation and internal thinking; for depth, you might decide you want to learn everything there is to learn about a topic you love; for joy, you might choose to jump on the trampoline with your child at the gym and have a serious laugh together. These feeling goals are powerful when combined with the body compass, where you sit still and check in with yourself to figure out if you really want to do something. For example, if you were invited to a group that discusses a favorite topic of yours, and adds an element of fun and grace, that group would speak to your feeling goals and it seems like attending it would be a huge yes. An invitation that leads you to a group that speaks negatively about others and brings you down would be a clear no. By making choices that support the way you want to feel, you'll be adding fuel back into your energy system instead of finding yourself depleted by choices that are incongruent with your values.

In the workbook will be a list of some feeling goals you can start playing around with, if you need some guidance. You'll probably want to have somewhere around three feeling goals at any given time. A fabulous resource to learn more on this general topic is Danielle LaPorte's *The Desire Map*, which brilliantly outlines a process to help you narrow down what she calls your Core Desired Feelings.

Humble goals are the next level of goals, external ones that are sort of like hobbies. Humble goals can be interrupted, compared to those bigger projects that require focus. A humble goal ideally fits within something you're passionate about, and would be one that you can easily do even with the interruption of small children—something you can pick up right where you left off, with minimal starting-power. These goals feed your understanding of yourself, and give you doses of reinforcement that you are still being you. I sat next to Edna on the buddy bench at my children's school the other week, watching the kids play on the playground while enjoying the last few days of warmth before winter kicked in. With her grey hair, colorful scarf, and light-catching dangling earrings, I wasn't entirely surprised to see she'd been knitting and, over the incredibly soft looking blanket, we started discussing what brought her to Denver and the various turns her life had taken. She talked to me about her identity as a passionate creative, how she'd met her husband at a Fine Arts program, and how they'd decided that they would always be involved in creative projects because that was what had brought them together and what made them the best versions of themselves. That was why she was currently knitting this blanket—this was her humble goal to fill the time gaps she had between watching her grandchild, one that brought her back to herself even for a few brief minutes. She said she was actually more of a painter, but she found herself frustrated with interruptions when working on a painting, so until she had the physical space and time in her new home to begin a bigger work, she would stick with other ways of feeling creative in small doses. Do you have any humble goals that spring to mind, from portable ones like knitting to more set ones like playing an instrument?

Edna also recommended enrolling in courses or programs that support your interests because, by putting money and investments into something, you're a lot more likely to get to that class and take the time to prioritize yourself. This could be a one-time course, like the one she was going to do the following week at the pottery studio, or an ongoing course that teaches you a bigger skill you want to learn for yourself. She observed that our generation was less inclined to take their hobbies seriously, but that hobbies offer such an important time out from the busy work of life, especially if those hobbies align with a passion, allowing for a rewarding connection with pleasure and a sense of self-nurturing. It continues to amaze me, as I look around at the people in our lives, how true this is—especially for women, who (admittedly a broad-brush observation) tend to be less likely to nurture their hobbies compared to men, who still go to play pickup basketball or brew beer in the garage. Kim pointed out to me once that the reason she continues to go to the horse stables (despite a busy husband and two small children and a separate Flex Mom goal she has for herself) is because horses are a passion of hers, something that she needs in her life to be a true, fulfilled version of herself. Perhaps some hobbies come and go, but they might stick around more if you spend some time figuring out which hobbies are in line with your passions. Then you will be much more likely to continue participating in that rejuvenating hobby, because you'll feel like the best, most true version of yourself.

"Big mama" goals are those that we set for longer stretches of time, those that a Flex Mom ultimately builds up to. These could be super long-term life goals, like becoming a professor at a prestigious university, or they could be more near-ish term life goals like publishing a book. Either way, they are projects that require planning and preparation and work over longer periods of time to achieve—but, BUT, they're achievable, even when you're raising children, because the process of achieving them fuels your fire. Some of you may know what your big mama goal is, because you've just always known. Others might not be sure yet what it is you want to achieve, and you'll spend some time thinking about it and revising this goal. To start the process, you'll want to grab a notebook and pen, and take time to be quiet. Call it your dream time, make yourself a cup of tea, turn off all computers and phones, put your feet up on the table, stare out the window and dream. What is it you'd love to do? If you were guaranteed success, what would you like to try? What makes you excited to think about accomplishing? What would you like people to remember you for? This is a huge brainstorm, so don't censor yourself—write down all the things that come to you in that happy dream state. You'll get to reevaluate later.

Feeling excited right now? That's awesome. Take a look back over that list of goals and figure out which ones make sense and still ring true in your real life, and which ones you're comfortable relegating to the "never" list (in my dream life I'd love to live in mainland China and learn the language, but given my real life, it's not a priority for me—it's better to move this off my brain to my "never" list than have it take up precious space in my mind). Then do a check-in with the next section to see if these goals fit the bill for meaningfulness—and if they do, you'll break the big mama goals into mini mama goals, to get you from here to where you want to be in a logical achievable sequence.

Pick Goals that are Meaningful: Rediscover Your Passions

One of the biggest concerns moms have at this stage is that they think they don't know what their passions are anymore. It's easy to believe that you have lost your passion because you have been deep into child rearing, that you've let yourself go for too long. It's intimidating to reflect back on who you used to be, because you're afraid you're not there anymore. But the thing is, passion is a strong desire, an emotion that motivates you to actually do something—it's something that is by definition meaningful to you. That sort of fire remains with us, deep inside, and it's a blast to explore it—especially when you discover how it has already come to manifest in your life as a parent.

It may seem like a daunting task to find your passion, so it will relieve you to know that it doesn't take a huge amount of effort. The easiest way is to find the answer to the question: "What do you find yourself doing even though you don't really have the time?"

For a college friend, Penelope, a corporate lawyer working crazy long hours, going to barre class was a normal thing for her. She'd had back surgery and wanted to continue strengthening her core, and it was a fabulous workout targeting all the areas she wanted. After the birth of her first child, she continued going to class, and was such a regular that she thought she might as well go through teacher training. So off she went, eventually starting to teach classes at 6am on Saturdays and even earlier once a week just so she could fit it in around her corporate work schedule—which, to an outsider, seems nuts to add into her life but was a source of sanity and strength for her. After the birth of her second child, she started reevaluating what she wanted to do, and eventually chose to leave her corporate law career and open up a barre studio so she could spend more time being with her family.

For Sarah, who I mentioned in the introduction, leaving her teaching career and being at home with her two children was the perfect opportunity to pursue her PhD—she figured, since she was home anyway, she might as well do something productive with that time. To an outsider, it would seem nuts to be reading and researching and missing extra sleep even when her two children were little, but to her, it was a goal worth pursuing as part of her bigger picture of continuing to be part of education and education policy. She would also say that the schoolwork and structure that provided was her sanity, her balancing act to the repetitions of parenting little ones. Now that her children are in school, she gets to spend time leading independent research studies in the public school system, largely thanks to that degree.

Your own passion is something that has probably always been within you, something that's always intrigued you, and that you could spend lots of time talking about or doing. For me, even when my children were little and always around, I continued to gravitate towards magazines and books and blogs on mind-body wellness and would read whenever I got a spare moment. As a parent, I had implemented tried and true positive psychology tricks to focus my family on scanning for the best parts of their day, and I modeled meditation and journaling with my girls. When I looked back, I realized I had strongly considered being a psychology major in college, and ended up taking several classes in the field; I was also always the person who friends sought out when they needed someone to talk things through with. I've been a life coach and wellness enthusiast my whole life.

If you're still unsure about your passion, about what it is you find meaningful, think about it in a much less lofty way—this is really a question that asks, "What is it that you want to do with your time, that is important to you?" Because you want to spend your precious time on things you feel are important! To explore this question further, there are several things you can do. Tap into your subconscious by free-associating what your ideal life might look like in five years. Grab a blank piece of paper (or a page in the workbook), write across the top "My ideal life in five years includes...." and imagine yourself at the age you will be five years into the future, imagine your children that age, imagine your partner and parents and siblings at that age. Then set a timer for two minutes and commit to writing continuously, uncensored, everything you think of—no matter how ridiculous it seems. Don't stop until the timer buzzes. When you are done, review your list, and circle the items that resonate the most with you—maybe eventually narrowing this list down to 5 to 10 key components.

Another data point in your exploration would be to think about what section you gravitate towards in a bookstore, or name the topics you feel so strongly about that you can meet a stranger and talk to them about with such focus that you lose your sense of time. To flip this exploration process on its head, you could also think about what lifestyle it is you want to create for yourself and for your family, spend time processing how it is you want to feel when you're pursuing this mysterious goal, and track backwards to see what things you care about that can fit into that ideal life. Mostly, though, reflect on what it is you're doing already that will give you clues about what you are passionate about.

The Intersection of Goals and Passion

Remember: passion is something that's already within you! And those goals that you dreamed about, those goals that you got excited about achieving, are so fun to pursue. To make your Flex Mom goal the most effective one, you want to find the intersection of your big mama goals and your passion. Yet, unless you have the right people around you to help bounce ideas around about what to do with that information, it's going to take time to find the best intersection of skills, passions, and desired lifestyle to find The Thing that you want to do with it.

You will probably set one goal, take steps towards achieving it, find a new path that branches from that path, and feel energized so long as these goals continue to be something that fuels your fire. For example, while I knew that sharing wellness was my passion, I didn't necessarily know what to do about it. Did I want to set up a coaching business (again)? Did I want to find a way to spread wellness through teaching? How could I set something up that would allow me to work during my kids' naptime or after bedtime, or during times that I hired support to have time for myself? I knew my longer-term vision was to be able to work during my kids' school day and still be able to pick them up, have summers off, and be flexible on all the random days off that come up during the school year—basically, being the Flex Mom without realizing it. With the support of my tribe, I was able to get on track pretty quickly. A friend from a non-profit board I was on wisely asked if I liked writing. Given that writing was the one thread I've had through all my careers, from writing about stock ideas to writing my coaching newsletters, it was a clear yes. She hooked me up with the team at a local mom's blog, and soon I found myself writing articles that related to my daily life as a mother. Within a short period of time, the team asked if I would manage the blog. This blogging was exactly the kind of thing I could do during naptime or after the kids' bedtimes, even dashing things off here and there when the children were driving me nuts and I put them in front of the TV—it fit my lifestyle. It was a great learning experience, and while it hadn't quite hit the mark in terms of intersecting with my wellness passions, it was great practice in writing and blogging and was in line with what I was enjoyed doing. My coach friend then emailed me the link to Angela Lauria's "The Author Incubator" program, which focuses on building a platform for coaches who want to positively influence our communities, and my whole body leaned toward the computer screen wondering how I could get accepted. This book, the very intersection of all of my interests and skills (wellness, writing, moms) came together in one beautiful vision. Be open to the series of "aha" moments in which the next step clicks into place, and if you can, build a support system that will encourage and challenge you, and point you in new possible directions so you don't have to feel isolated in the process of finding the goal that's best for you.

If you operate visually and want a way to see the passion and goal setting process, picture it as a Trim a Home® lighted spiral tree, where one string of lights circles widely around the bottom and continues to curve around in ever tightening spirals all the way up until it reaches the bright star at the very top. You'll go around and around experimenting, trying on new things, and feeling like you're moving in the right direction and that the answer you're looking for is right around the corner. Getting support from the right sources—a coach, a highly observant and honest friend—will accelerate this process of identifying your passion. You will then come around the last bend and it'll all crystalize in that one fine point, a bright shiny star. This passionate goal that you set will leave you feeling a sense of joy and relief and excitement. This will be your parallel track to your hamster wheel, the thing that helps define you outside of your child-rearing, the thing that makes you a Flex Mom. Once it's identified, you'll come up with a plan, breaking the achievement of that big mama goal into mini mama goals, so you can move forward to achieve them instead of letting them just sit in the back of your brain.

If you're reading this during your first year of parenthood, when it's all about survival—no matter whether you work or stay at home—when your life is dominated by making it through sleepless nights and feeding patterns and diaper changes and adjusting your whole world view, please don't feel you have to master this part of the program. If you feel you have the capacity, absolutely go ahead and start brainstorming and moving forward with articulating your passions and taking some next steps. If it's too much for you to make extra commitments because of all the moving parts involved in this stage of parenting, give yourself time to regroup, work on building up those foundational habits of a healthy Flex Mom, and relaunch the process of identifying your goals once your children are in the toddler years and you have a bit more independence again!

CHAPTER 6
EXAMINE YOUR BOUNDARIES

"Daring to set boundaries is about having the courage to love ourselves, even when we risk disappointing others."
—Brené Brown

When we were still living in Arizona and looking for our first home, we came across a foreclosure that we thought we liked. The markets were not doing particularly well, and it was clear that the realtor we had been working with was pulling out all the stops to make the pieces fit together to close the deal so she could get paid. A week or so into working with this realtor on the house, it was becoming apparent that we were not going to get the place, but she still kept us for multiple extra hours at the house to try "just one more thing." Soon it was 6pm, and she was stressfully juggling conversations with her daughter, who had come home from school hours earlier and was needing her mom, with conversations with the bank and the mortgage companies that we were working with. Meanwhile, John and I sat twiddling our thumbs, leaning against the kitchen countertops with nothing to do but again be told to sit and wait and be ignored while she frantically tried to close this deal in a very slow market. Her daughter continued to call and text, and eventually, as the clock ticked straight through dinnertime, we said we'd had enough and that we were walking away. She clearly disappointed her daughter AND she didn't get business done—mostly because she was so distracted and unclear with us about the process that we finally got fed up and were willing to lose the house.

Without establishing your boundaries to begin with, without defining what you stand for and what you need to make those things happen, you will end up feeling frustrated, disconnected, and, most likely, lonely. To keep your daily management of the children and home afloat, and to have enough support to pursue your passion project, it's important for you, as a Flex Mom, to define certain boundaries. These boundaries will protect the time you need to prioritize being present for your family and to move forward with your goals. The boundaries you want to examine are around your technology usage, your time, and your community.

How and Why to Set Your Technology Boundaries

My husband and I are slightly more old school when it comes to family values and, especially given how much he travels, we make a point of enjoying quality conversation with the kids whenever we can. One day after school, my oldest daughter sat down at the kitchen island for some snacks and, within a few minutes, said to me, "Mom, can you please just put your phone down already? You're always on that thing." I'd always prided myself on being consciously disconnected when the kids were around, but without realizing it, I'd picked up my phone when a text from my brother came in talking about a family issue and I had been starting a dialogue with him. I thought I'd put my phone down between texts and made eye contact with my daughter, but she knew I was distracted. And she was right—a recent study showed that both parties rated a conversation as less satisfactory when a cell phone was simply visibly placed on the table, versus placed out of sight in a purse or in a different room. My daughter called me on our need to clearly define our tech boundaries in the house, because even for someone who is aware of that downside, it was easy for me to slip up and make her feel less important and less connected to her family.

There are any number of ways to define your tech boundaries. One is to think about creating a "tech-free zone" or a "no-phone zone." One family decided that they would never allow any technology at the dinner table—even for mom or dad, who were known until that point to take "just this one message about work" during their moments together. They decided to set the tone for the family because they didn't want their kids to do the same thing to them when they were old enough to have their own phones. Another family does not allow technology on the living room sofa, even when the whole extended family is gathered there chatting after a Thanksgiving meal and is tempted to look at the latest shopping deals and check in with friends. It forces them to sit and actually have conversation, and often means that they get into deeper, juicier topics because they aren't tempted by the pull of technology to opt out of the interactions. For us, after my daughter's comments, we created a charging station in the area just off the kitchen, where all of our cell phones live when we are not using them. It makes it impossible to fool yourself into thinking you're participating in family discussion when you have to get up and walk to a different area to pick up a text. In fact, my friends and family know that if they want to reach me urgently, they need to actually call me because I won't pick up a text when I'm chatting or playing with my kids, or if I'm in the middle of a project. This setup helps protect me from distraction and gives me the space to actually focus on my priorities.

Learn to Prioritize Your Time

Veronica is a married-yet-effectively-single mom with two children and a husband who travels loads for work. She finds that the time when her husband is on the road drags, stretching out and seeming like forever—and yet during those stretches, her energy also flags, so she rarely feels like she has time to take a shower and clean up after meals, let alone make time to finish editing the photos she's been working on for the last few months. Her perpetual complaint was, "I don't have time!" and she was finding it frustrating to be stuck without forward momentum. Veronica's breakthrough happened when she realized she needed to accept that her life wouldn't necessarily be consistent, and that she could carve out time when it worked in her life—that is, ask for support when her husband was home, ask a neighbor for a kid swap, find an older neighbor to be a "mothers helper"—to get an hour during the day to sit at her computer and work on catching up on the day to day and get herself started on her images. She also realized that she wasn't making the most of her night owl tendencies. She discovered that if she set her children's bedtime just 30 minutes earlier, not only would the mornings go more smoothly, with happier children, but she could transition into having some alone time to recharge, giving herself enough energy to claim over an hour of productive time before she went to sleep. In fact, her problem became that she was getting so sucked into her project, in that flow state, that she would be up until the wee hours of the morning if she wasn't careful!

Time boundaries help to make us more mindful of the time we do have, and make us aware of the time we don't use effectively. When we know what our own cycles are—like Veronica did when she capitalized on those evening hours—and we decide what our potential routines can be, our brains relax into knowing that we have protected time to let our creativity flow. Think about when it is that you work best, and when you might have or can create some protected time, and see how you can arrange your schedule to support those blocks of time for your own work. Be conscious of what you want to achieve, and find the time for it to happen regularly.

In addition to thinking about time to work, be sure that you're blocking out time for things that are important to maintaining your sense of self. If you find that you are an introvert and need alone time to recharge, plot that into your day or your evening—a bubble bath, a magazine by the fire, a float in the pool, a quick walk around the block after the kids are asleep. This isn't a luxury, but a necessary part of self-maintenance, so don't second guess yourself—make it a priority to make that alone time happen. If you enjoy date nights or conversation time with your partner, figure out with what frequency you need these dates to happen and carve out the easiest way to make them happen. For my husband and me, we don't need to go out to dinner very often because we cook great meals at home with the family, but we do enjoy a nightcap on our front porch at night, often in lieu of our favorite TV shows.

If you want to catch up with your friends—and social networks are one of the most important things for your health and happiness—find ways to incorporate those interactions in your life more regularly. You can plan to bring the kids to a group exercise class and connect with moms, you can host survival dinners where you serve whatever you have in the fridge for dinner and have a glass of wine with a friend while the kids play together, you can join a book club and make those dates iron-clad in your calendar. Know that some moms go dark and hermit-like when they're having a tough time, and that what you need to snap out of it is exactly what you're not doing—connecting with people. Even while you are busy pursuing your goals, find what frequency of social interaction works for you, and make the time in your life to commit to those events and your important relationships, because the daily busy work of life will often expand into your day if you do not consciously carve the time out.

Keep in mind that boundaries are most certainly important, but when they get blurred—especially with small children in the picture—it will make life go more smoothly when you don't judge too harshly (see: no judging!), when you don't get too upset that things aren't panning out exactly the way you'd hoped. Case in point: all parents want to use the restroom without interruption. Yet, most days, little feet come and barge in through the door, talking to you about the cool pattern they made using their new crayons, or what food they just spilled on the floor. In my case, the best moment was when I excused myself from the kitchen and thought I'd escaped while the children were distracted. The next thing I know, I hear "knock knock knock-knock knock," followed by a whiny melody: "Do you wanna build a snooowwwwwmannnnn?" When I remained silent, albeit with a smirk on my face, my daughter repeated the knocking and singing, and demanded that I reply. Next thing you know, I found myself singing "I hardly see you anymore" and doing my part in a line-by-line reenactment of that famous scene from "Frozen." A much more humorous result than being frustrated yet again, despite not getting the brief time alone that I wanted.

Carve Out a Supportive Community to Meet Your Goals

Joanna is an American woman who married a Spanish man and is raising their multi-cultural children in Madrid. As many people do in a mid-city apartment unit, they live amid hundreds of other families in the complex, and she explained how easy it is to feel more relaxed about work and home because she has the support of all of her neighbors-turned-supporters. It's a common thing for her children to go downstairs to the community pool and be watched by the neighbors while she makes dinner; she would do the same in a heartbeat for all of her neighbor's children. The concept of "it takes a village" is played out in many other parts of the world—but often, with our isolated homes and garage door syndrome (where we close the garage door as soon as we pull our car in, before we even step out), our community resources are left untapped in the United States.

How difficult do you find it to ask your neighbor to watch your child so you can dash off to the doctor's office, without feeling like you need to offer them something in exchange? How easy is it for you to send the kids to ring the doorbell of a friend's house to invite themselves to play, or have kids just stop by your home and let them come in for an hour or two, at the last minute? These interactions nowadays are pretty scripted and awkward, pre-arranged by text or email often weeks in advance, even though deep in our hearts we might want to have flowing homes filled easily with people who stop by and would do the same for us.

The Harvard Grant study followed men for 75 years and showed that the depth and breadth of relationships these men had were some of the biggest predictors of their longevity and health and happiness. And anybody who has read Malcolm Gladwell's *Outliers* knows that even Bill Gates did not achieve his success in a vacuum—it was a confluence of events and people and access that allowed him to get the experience he needed to set up and dominate through Microsoft. Our community plays a huge role in shaping who we are, and who we can be. It would appear we need to reevaluate, reengage and reclaim the people we surround ourselves with.

Where do you start? First, you want to think about your people. Your real people, people who will help support your goals. To be conscious of where you are, my old coaching clients found it helpful to do a conscious revamp of the people in their lives. I remember being inspired years ago by something in Cheryl Richardson's book *Take Time for your Life*. By listing out different categories, like kids and mom friends and acquaintances and career support and real friends and family and spiritual support, and brain dumping everyone you know into one of these categories—making sure that they only fit into one or another—you can get a snapshot of where you stand. Is your list balanced the way that you want it to be? What categories are overflowing, and which are lacking? Then, take a look at those individuals in the list that sort of give you the blahs—are there people on the list that don't really lift you up, who kind of drain you, who you find annoying to be around? Cross them off the list, with the intention of slowly removing their presence from your lives. Don't feel badly—nobody will see this list and you don't have to come back to it again. But, for your sake, cross them off. Now take a look at individuals on the list who you think might be better served in one category instead of the one they're listed in. I have a friend, Jaime, who was an acquaintance, but I knew would make a spectacular addition to my spiritual community and, within a month of circling her name and moving it under the spiritual list, we connected in a different, even deeper way than we had before. So go ahead and circle those people, and pull their names to their new category. Take a few minutes to reflect on this list, review the names, and realize that your community is way richer than you'd probably known before you wrote it all down. And once it's done, feel free to thank the universe and burn this list, or shred it, or toss it in the recycling—or keep it tucked away for comparison when you do this exercise again in a year.

Now that you know who your people are, it's time to articulate who your helpers are. What are the things you need to do to maintain the standards you want for your family? Do you manage to clean the bathrooms and vacuum the house and dust the furniture effortlessly, or could you use some help? Are you happy with how your family is fed? Are you getting the exercise and sleep that you want? Beyond that, what is the space you need to have to not just survive motherhood, but thrive by adding your Flex Mom component? Do you have several hours per week to dedicate to your own passion? What would you need to do to get that time? Do you have people to bounce your ideas around with, to give you the juice and feedback you need to keep pushing forward? The standard rule of thumb is to figure out what help it is you need to get by, and then add to it—because you will need more support than you think you need.

For many parents, getting help to do a deep clean of the house is a fabulous place to start for support. While I managed to make the kitchen clean and sanitary by the end of each day, and managed to clean the toilets and bathrooms while my children were in the baths, I didn't always (all right, ever) get around to deep cleaning the refrigerator each month, or dusting the unseen high corners of the cabinets. Asking for support by hiring housecleaners every few weeks freed up both mental and physical time for me to channel into my work. If that's not within your budget, find a way to make it a game and involve the rest of the family, so you are spending time together instead of building up resentment that you have to do it all alone.

To get time to yourself, many people who are lucky enough to have extended family living close by enlist the help of grandparents, aunties, or uncles. Your relatives get to have special bonding time with your little people, your children get the benefit of developing deep relationships with adults aside from you and your partner, and you get some time to recharge your batteries. If you (like me) don't have any extended family nearby, you can build out your babysitter list, so instead of relying on one person's availability, you have a deeper roster of support. By the time my second child was a couple of years old, my husband and I agreed that it made sense to hire a sitter once a week for me to get stuff like errands done without hauling two kids in and out of the car each time, or to have an uninterrupted lunch date with a new inspirational person, and mostly to have a stretch of time to let my brain run free. If babysitting isn't in the budget, initiate with some friends a weekly kid-swap, where you watch your friend's children once a week for several hours at a time, and then they agree to watch your children for several hours at a time. You may find a hidden benefit, that the children play together so well that they will require less of your attention than if you were simply spending time with your own children—so you get two-ish chunks of time per week to do your own thing.

For your goals, build out a personal Board of Directors, people who you trust to give you honest, direct feedback and be some of your biggest cheerleaders for success. Who are some people who initially spring to mind for you? These people can be friends, old colleagues, acquaintances you admire—but mostly they are people who motivate you and inspire you and teach you. If, for example, Veronica was to build out her Board of Directors to expand her photography business, she wouldn't just ask another photographer friend with her exact same set of starting skills— she would look for a variety of people, including someone who could represent a potential client, a fellow Flex Mom who could offer moral support, someone with an expertise in financial matters, a professional photographer with a successful business. When you get stuck or have a question about what you're doing, your Board members are the first people you turn to for advice. These people know that you think highly of them, and you do what you can to support them in return.

Having examined your community and rules around how you manage your time and technology, you should be feeling a lot more connected and inspired by the space you have to pursue your goal. Imagine yourself no longer on a deserted island drowning in a sea of used baby diapers, and instead imagine yourself as the hub on a spoked wheel, directing that bicycle towards your goals.

CHAPTER 7
MINDFULNESS

"Life is what happens on the way to the finish line."
—Danielle LaPorte

Remember when your child was just starting to eat, and decided that he loved bananas, and would eat them every single day with gusto? You couldn't get enough bananas at the store to feed this child. He would have a full one each night before bed as a snack, after already having had one at breakfast. The bananas would never get a chance to go fully ripe, and you'd have to get to the store several times a week just to stock the kitchen. Until suddenly, with no warning, he wouldn't eat bananas. Would clamp his mouth shut and turn his head away, smacking the thing away, and suddenly you were stuck with a month's worth of frozen bananas to blend into your smoothies.

Just when you think you've figured life out, things will change. Just when you think you've got this Flex Mom thing down pat, things will change.

It can be pretty paralyzing to go from thinking you have things figured out, when you're in the flow of working towards your goal, and then having what feels like a huge stop sign right in front of you. But that is life, and a Flex Mom takes that "stop" sign and reads it as a "yield" sign instead. To better deal with a shape-shifting life, you want to be aware of things, knowing and sensing the big picture and the potential knock-on effects of any changes—which, without judging where you are, will help you to be open to many more options when life throws you a curveball. These skills are part of the bigger movement called mindfulness.

In a Flex Mom's life, these skills are very useful when, for example, you're working on your passion project, preparing to conduct an interview, and your eldest child develops a fever and has to stay home sick from school. Instead of getting all angry and judgmental and wallowing in the tough situation you're in, instead of only seeing the black or white option of going alone or cancelling the interview, you quickly think of an alternative. You note that your child is feeling pretty mellow, isn't vomiting or having to be chained to a toilet, so is definitely mobile—and so you get to that interview by bringing your kid along with a blanket, Tylenol, tissues, and iPad. You can go with the flow, because you're observing and open to different options to get the same result.

Mindfulness Skill 1: Single-Tasking

In our busy world, a major step towards mindfulness is to switch from multi-tasking to single-tasking. When you are busy doing more than one thing at a time, something that us moms are well accomplished in doing, your brain isn't being trained to focus well. Witness us running around like chickens with our heads cut off, looking for that set of keys that we swore we put down on top of our purse when little Johnny was crying and you were trying to catch the shoes that his big sister was throwing across the room at his head while you were finishing up a phone call with your own mother, so you don't quite remember where those darn keys are. You weren't really paying attention to where you put those keys because you were doing a lot at once.

If you are skeptical about the power of single-tasking and want more proof, just look at my favorite study about humans driving a (simulated) car while talking on a phone. The results of the functional MRI showed that listening and understanding language actually took your brainpower away from the act of driving—meaning, you had both a worse quality conversation and were a worse driver when you did both at once. This study proved to the researchers that the brain physically cannot multi-task. It actually has a limited capacity and, instead of truly multi-tasking, it switches between two tasks rapidly, with neither task getting the full capacity that it would get if each was done alone. Really, multi-tasking is a myth, and we perform at much better capacity if we do one thing at a time.

Did you hear that? We perform much better if we do one thing at a time. It explains why Nicole found her coffee mug in the microwave, cold yet again, day after day, until she realized that she would enjoy the mornings a lot more by shifting her priorities and letting the kids watch one television show each morning after breakfast and getting dressed, just so she could take a few moments to make herself a fresh cup and sit still and enjoy a blissfully uninterrupted 15 minutes to drink the hot coffee.

This translates into the world of being a Flex Mom because of course, having children, we are already very used to getting multiple things done at once. Imagine how much more efficient and effective we would be if we focused on getting one thing done at a time! As we make a conscious effort to practice our single-tasking skills, doing one thing at a time—especially during the times when we are doing things for ourselves—we will become even more effective in reaching our goals because we will be performing at peak capacity.

For any mothers who have said they feel dumber by being a mom, you are not alone. I can relate firsthand to this notion of feeling dumber, because even though I joined a high power organization after graduating from Harvard, I could have sworn that, with the hundreds of daily emails and constant shrill of phone calls and multiple conversations going at once, I was finding it harder to come up with the right words I needed on the spot. And then, once I had kids and got peppered by their regular interruptions, I could have sworn that my brain cells were simply transferred out of my body at birth, because there was no way that I could complete a crossword puzzle anymore (not even a Monday edition). Turns out all of our instincts are right. Distraction makes us duller.

Studies have shown that people who are heavy multi-taskers of media are much more susceptible to irrelevant distractions from the environment and have irrelevant representations in their memory. This, surprisingly to the researchers, meant that these multi-taskers performed worse in their ability to switch tasks, compared to those who are low multi-taskers. So for those of us who are constantly interrupting ourselves by compulsively checking emails and Facebook and of course getting interrupted by the "Mom, I'm hungry" cries, we are not maximizing our potential. Which is why when we have the opportunity, especially when we are working on our passion-goal, it's important for us to practice single-tasking.

Besides, if we do one thing at a time, we are more likely to be aware of what is influencing our mood or our capacity. Using mindfulness to observe what's going on is a cool trick, as it lets us step out of our instinct to react and instead encourages us to respond—much like the skills of "the pause" and deep breathing let us do (you'll learn more about this in the next chapter). We are watching ourselves from outside, observing the things that are going on both inside and outside of our bodies, without judgment. And that is crucial, to let yourself simply be and observe what's going on instead of berating yourself for the situation that you're in or the feelings that you're having.

Mindfulness Skill 2: Still Time

Another way mindfulness can be applied is simply to take time, sort of like the time outs we give children. It's okay to give ourselves time outs as well. I use this method when my kids aren't behaving in a way I want them to, and I notice that my own heart is beating faster and I'm feeling steam building up inside of me. This doesn't happen as often as it used to, but on some occasions—especially when I'm sleep deprived—my patience isn't what it normally is and I get more frustrated. Instead of telling the kids that they're in trouble, I tell them that mommy needs a time out, time to go cool off and be by myself so I can treat them more kindly when I get out. I don't go far, but I do give myself some stillness in a corner of the house somewhere. This feels a lot better than waiting until after I've exploded and I sit hiding on the floor of my closet crying in shame because I just had way worse self-control than a three-year-old would have had.

You don't have to wait until after you're in a heated situation to give yourself this time out. Sitting in silence, sitting still, is a practice we can incorporate even during a regular day. The next time you're out for food and your dining partner gets up from the table during a meal, don't grab your phone—sit in the silence and look around at the other diners. The next time you've arrived a few minutes early to school pick up, step outside the car and walk around, breathing in the fresh air. Create space and stillness in your daily life, and you'll be surprised at the benefits. You may be inspired by a new thought, or a new goal, and get a new "aha" moment about the things you want to accomplish in your own life.

The main difference my friend Alex noticed when she incorporated more still time into her life was that she had space to suddenly do the things that she wanted to do. Instead of running around doing one thing after another, she found that as she had these pockets of time, she was able to make that unplanned phone call to an inspirational friend, or plan a coffee with an old colleague to talk about the fashion world she was interested in getting into. These connections fueled her energy and kept her inspired to work towards her goal. Even though she then did get a little bit busier, she knew she was on the right track because she felt more energized by these purposeful plans and interactions than she had by the busywork with which she had previously been filling her time.

Mindfulness Skill 3: Reframing

My younger child is the best person I have met to exemplify the benefits of reframing. When she was little and barely able to string sentences together, it was raining and I felt stuck. It was just about dinner prep time, and sending her outside to play meant she'd probably get muddy and would need me to help wash up just as I was cooking. I said as much, sighing about the weather, and she perked up, "It's okay Mommy, after the rain we get to see RAINBOWS!" Another time, our good family friend had a mother who passed away, and as I spoke with her on speakerphone, I saw my youngest grabbing for the handset. She proudly proclaimed, "Auntie, I'm sorry your mommy died. But she's going to be okay, she can go have a play date with my grandpa now!" That sort of sounds like innocent optimism, but it really is a method of reframing.

Reframing is a way to look at the same situation and interpret it in a more positive way. Many people who are faced with really difficult situations tend to default to this, if they are primed to be more positive. It was devastating when my father passed away, but shortly after the fact, we moved away from boo-hooing about it and instead, verbalized that if such a kind person was going to have to die, at least he died relatively quickly and had a solid three weeks when we were able to say goodbye to him. Or, when the husband of a woman I worked with was attacked in a bar, a bottle smashed over his head that cut his eye, she came to our call apologizing for being late, saying that they were so lucky that it was only one eye that was damaged, and that there was still hope for him to return to driving again. She could have felt very sorry for herself, and for him, wondering "why him?"—but instead, she reframed it by saying it could have been much worse.

This skill of reframing turns setbacks into positive challenges. My coach during this book process insightfully said that every author encounters challenges to the writing process—a sudden surgery that needs to take place, a roof leak that destroys part of a home and requires repairs, a fun anniversary trip that has been planned for months that takes place shortly before the deadline. Some people might use those challenges as an excuse not to meet goals, wallowing in a bit of self-pity and hardship, saying just how tough it was to keep on going. Instead, coach Angela expected us to be the person who got the book done *despite* all of those challenges, to be the person who could say, "Can you believe that I got this book done even though I had appendicitis and had to go through emergency surgery?" What a powerful reframing process. So when the same happens to you during your process of pursuing your passion project, change your perspective to be the person who got things done despite all the challenges along the way. Because you want to be that person, that Flex Mom who is flexible and will adapt to the circumstances that will inevitably shift and try to stand in the way of you achieving your goals.

To cement this notion of mindfulness, visualize being an invisible friend hovering around listening to and observing what's going on in your life. That friend is your cheerleader, your supporter, and the person who wants to be able to communicate with you. Slow down the chatter in your life so you can make space for that friend, to listen to her neutral observations as she helps you to see challenges in ways that can be solved.

CHAPTER 8
OPEN YOUR MOUTH WISELY

"Speak clearly, if you speak at all; carve every word before you let it fall."
—Oliver Wendell Holmes, Sr.

My youngest child started a full-day kindergarten program this fall. Until that day, I had had someone by my side for about 12 hours a day for seven years in a row. On that first day of school, there were tears of joy (and a little nostalgia, sure), mostly for the celebratory culmination of Parenting Phase 1. With both of my girls now in school full time, I was thrilled to be entering what I consider Parenting Phase 2, with more than six hours a day to myself, five days a week. After a week of mani-pedis and massages to pamper myself for years of stay-at-home parenting well survived, I had set myself up to start writing this book. I was overjoyed at the prospect of working on this goal that I'd set for myself, and still being able to be there for the kids when they got home from school. Every day, I came home from drop-off, made myself a cup of coffee, sat down to the laptop, and got to work.

About an hour into it each day, as I wandered back into the kitchen to get myself a glass of water or another cup of coffee, I frowned at the dirty dishes sitting on the counter. Why the heck do I have to do the *dishes* when I'm an important author-in-transformation working on my book? I have a career in the making, and I have to be bothered with home-making work?? Then I'd look at the laundry upstairs and realize that yet again, I'd left the wet clothes sitting in the machine, now smelling a bit moldy and in need of just one more run through the wash. But I didn't want to spend the time on it.

My ever-supportive husband, when he was home between trips, would do the laundry he hated doing to give me some space and time to work, leaving it nicely folded in each room. It was only when he got home from five days away and the folded laundry was still sitting there, not put away, that we had a reality check. Writing a book does not mean that the rest of our home would magically be taken care of by someone else. Either I needed to find a way to moderate my schedule or we needed to hire a daily housekeeper. We recalibrated—okay, I recalibrated—back to our originally stated family values and roles and found a better compromise.

It wasn't that he was expecting me to be a housekeeper. He was expecting me to continue doing my share to keep the house running, just like any other person who lives with other people, whether they work or stay at home. I had just developed a resentful attitude because, after years of "sacrificing" my time to be present for the children and doing my part to run the household, I was finally doing things for myself and wanted nothing to get in my way.

I had figured out the whole Flex Mom theory and was super excited to put it into action, so I developed a little resentment towards my husband because, much as he does more than his share of things around the house when he's home, much as he was supportive about the idea of me writing this book, I wasn't feeling like he understood that I just wanted to rid myself of all responsibilities and do what I wanted. Which, of course, wasn't realistic. Still, resentment can creep its ugly little head into many aspects of life—and nothing is more harmful than when resentment slips into a marriage and home. If you don't catch it early enough, resentment morphs into contempt, and according to John Gottman, contempt is the single greatest predictor of divorce. And that was not what I wanted, so we hashed it out.

If, through reading this book, you've decided that you are interested in becoming a Flex Mom, you will want to loop your partner into a conversation and begin discussing what it is you envision, just like you did when you decided to become a stay-at-home mother. You'll want to explain to your partner all the benefits of becoming a Flex Mom instead of a stay-at-home mom—the excitement and fulfillment you'll feel pursuing your passion, the energy that will flow back to your family, the interesting conversations you can have with your partner about your goals, and the role model you can be for your children as you show them that it's okay for you to pursue your own happiness. You'll also want to open the door to talking about what concerns you and your partner about becoming a Flex Mom, and how you can best pursue your passions while continuing to honor your family. I'm going to bet that my husband isn't the only partner who doesn't love dramatic, unannounced change. Maybe you start by leaving a copy of this book lying around in obvious places, where it might spark conversation. Maybe you mention how happy so-and-so is, who started doing this Flex Mom thing. In any case, you will want to open your mouth wisely to communicate your desire to shake things up a bit on the home front.

Here are some of the best communication tools you can rely on, both for this initial conversation and to continue holding space for your passion as challenges arise.

Communication Skill 1: Using "I Statements"

Going back to the laundry challenges in our house during the writing of the book, would it have been helpful for me to respond to John defensively, saying, "Most authors need to create lots of space in their lives, you know, to be creative, so it's your problem that it bothers you that I didn't get around to putting the laundry away—you have a few days off now, so why don't you do it?" Nope, that would have seriously pissed him off and the whole conversation would have spiraled out of control. Instead, one of the first things I used was "I statements."

I explained how I was feeling, literally using the words "I" and "feelings." I was feeling resentful not about him in particular, but about this idea that after all these years of sacrificing myself for the kids, it was my time to do something for myself and I didn't want to give an inch. That I realized that this approach was unrealistic and selfish, and that I needed help figuring out a plan to make both writing and home-making work because I didn't like feeling resentful. Phrased in this way, John could hear my concerns without feeling defensive. The great thing about using "I statements" is that the person listening can't really argue with what you say, because you are stating how you feel, something that is true to you, and you're not making any accusations. In doing so, you create an opportunity to share your feelings and perspectives without your partner feeling that they are in the wrong.

Perhaps when you're having your initial transition into Flex Mom conversation, you might say, "I was really excited about staying at home to raise the children, because they are so important to me, and this family is so important to me. I've found that the reality of staying at home isn't the same as what I'd expected—I'm a lot more drained and lonely than I anticipated, and I'm afraid my negativity is wearing onto the kids and maybe even us. I am thinking about ways to make this a better experience for me, and for the kids, and for all of us..."

Communication Skill 2: Active Listening

In response to my "I statements" about laundry, John explained what he'd been noticing. Instead of jumping in and defending myself when he commented on something that I didn't like about myself (I hate being told I'm not living up to expectations, even if it is about laundry), I used another tactic. I did not interrupt. Nope, no interruptions. I just held space for him to say everything he needed to say, nothing but a nod of agreement here or there, or a non-verbal murmur to show him I was still listening. Not only does not interrupting give the person talking a sense of respect, a sense that they are being listened to, but it gives the person listening time to actually listen, without feeling the compulsion to give in to that knee-jerk reaction to say something in return. This is called active listening—where you want to get to the root of the problem, deeply listening even to what's not being said, to understand what it is the speaker is really trying to communicate.

It turns out that John wasn't upset so much about the laundry itself, but about this sense that I was suddenly shifting from a person who did everything for the house to someone who did nothing for the house, and it was disconcerting to him because he wasn't sure how to handle this new person. He never said those words out loud, but given that my husband is a man who doesn't like too much change—he's a pilot, this is a good and expected thing, a man who operates with checklists and all that—I could hear it in the undertones of what he was saying. I had my mind open and left the silent space where I didn't interrupt, and I was actively listening for what he wasn't saying. Then, I gathered my thoughts so I could respond positively, because suddenly he morphed from an annoying person who was on my case about a folded pile of laundry to a man I love who doesn't like change and doesn't want his wife to become a different person overnight.

Communication Skill 3: The Pause

Before responding to John's feedback, I just took a deep breath. That's all it takes sometimes to keep the tone of the conversation positive, moving in a productive direction. The same way that you take a deep breath, maybe even count to 10, before you lose your cool on the kid who accidentally shattered the bowl of cereal and milk on the floor because they didn't clear the dishes the way you told them to, this deep breath works for adult conversations as well. You go from "How many times do I have to tell you to get off the stinkin' chair FIRST and THEN get your bowl down from the table, don't you ever listen to me?!" to "Honey, I appreciate that you were being responsible by clearing your dishes, but do you understand now why I say to get off the chair first instead of grabbing the dishes first? Please don't do it again. Now help me clean this mess up."

Together, we realized that if we/I just spent 30 minutes a day on house-related things (aside from cooking dinner), then we had tidied up and taken care of almost everything that had been causing friction before. Now, if we weren't constantly working on our communication skills, this tension could have built up and led to a much bigger, more devastating conversation that could have derailed my plans and desire to write this book—all over some ridiculous belief I had developed that I didn't have to do anything around the house anymore.

Communication Skill 4: Using Your NO Muscle

All of the skills above are incredibly useful when communicating with your partner both during the initial transition to being a Flex Mom, and as challenges come up during the process of pursuing your goals. This next skill, while also applicable in your relationship, is most important for you to use to create and hold space for your priorities—especially your Flex Mom goals. It is the skill of saying no.

When my friend Anna and I chatted about this idea of saying no, she was a mom overrun by a life largely run solo, with a busy husband, multiple birthday party invitations each weekend, kids' activities nearly every afternoon of the week and most weekends, and her own desire to go out for girls' nights and book clubs and drinks with friends. If one hiccup happened—a flat tire, a kid being sick—the domino effects were tremendous, so she fretted about every eventuality and was regularly stressed out about doing it all. She would be invited to yet another thing, and even if she didn't want to go, she'd reply "maybe" thinking that, if only the stars aligned just right, she would be able to make it to that event.

This fear of missing out happens to everyone, but realize what this is—it's simply living in fear. Making decisions based on fear is an exhausting way to operate, because it usually involves making choices based on other people's values and expectations. The reason we spent so much time earlier in this process working on outlining your values and desires is just for this situation—to arm you with the confidence that you know yourself and know what works for you, and to know that you can say no to things that don't work. We need to be able to say no to clear space for the things and lifestyle we want to say yes to. Please remember that saying no, that choosing what you want to do instead of what you think is expected of you, does not make you a bad person. It doesn't make you selfish or unkind.

How do you know the difference between what you want to say yes to and no to? You listen to your body. This is why we talked about making sure your body is getting enough sleep, exercise, and sensuality to be optimally primed to move forward. The conscious verbal mind can process approximately 40 bits of information per second; the subconscious mind processes multiple magnitudes more information than the conscious—the estimates range from 11-40 *million* bits of info per second. You need to be in touch with your body to listen to what your subconscious has to say to you regarding decisions you want to make, because it can tell you so much more than your brain can often articulate. The way to understand the difference between a yes and a no is that making decisions out of fear (saying yes when you really want to say no) will feel like dread. If you close your eyes and imagine the thing that you are deciding about, if you sit still and tune into your body, you might find yourself physically leaning back away from that thing, maybe feeling a drag somewhere in your body. On the opposite side of the spectrum, you know when you are saying yes to things that light your fire, things that you love and are important to you, because it feels uplifting and freeing. If you tune into your body, if you can imagine that decision or thing, you will be leaning in. When I heard about this book-writing program, despite being terrified about committing to something big and knowing the cost involved, I found myself practically face to face with the computer screen with excitement because I knew I was all in, and my body was screaming yes. Your body is a powerful tool and will help you in making decisions that best work for you, so cherish it and listen when it guides you.

To give yourself the space and mental energy you'll need to pursue your goals and passions as Flex Moms, it's important to say no to things that you don't want to do. Once you've tuned into your body to understand what really floats your boat and what makes you shrink back, it's important to translate that into actually saying what you mean. Time spent on events that aren't in line with your values can sap your energy. So if the invitation for another birthday party comes in the mail and you really don't like the kid or the parents, say no. If you get invited for drinks on a Friday but you know that by that stage in the week you will really just want to take a long soak in the bathtub to treat yourself to a night of quiet pampering after the kids are in bed, say no. OR, if you want to desperately socialize with adults and want to change those plans you made with yourself to soak in a tub, say no to the tub and go on out. The key is to use "the pause" and tune into what it is you really want to do, and communicate your desires clearly. People—including your partner—will not be offended if you say no with the best intentions. If they invite you out, politely decline with a kind thank you for the invitation. No need for excuses, just be sincere!

One major communication slip that people often make is saying "maybe," when that's not what they really mean. Of course there are times when that's really the answer you want to give, but it's important to realize that "maybe" is often just a softer way of saying "no." Did you really think that that friend whose kid was up all night and whose husband is traveling, who said "maybe" when you invited her out for drinks, is really going to come out? No, deep in her heart she probably meant no, but didn't feel comfortable saying it. Please, take the time to figure out what you want, and then say what you mean. If you say it with the best intentions, people will understand and know that you are a woman of integrity and are doing what is best for you.

When Anna finally started saying no to extra things—when she started saying no to renewing the kids' extracurricular activities that they weren't enjoying, when she said no to the invitations out for a second book club since she knew she would never read the books—she found she actually had time to reconnect with her husband on more date nights (which she wanted), and she had time and more energy to focus on developing her own passion.

Communication Skill 5: Being Aware of Your Non-Verbal Cues

I can't let a chapter on communication skills go without mentioning what can be the most impactful but least discussed method of communication—our body language and tone of voice. When there is a discrepancy between what your words are saying and how your body is acting, your body language is actually the thing that's going to get its message across more clearly. In this context, according to UCLA researcher Albert Mehrabian, body language is more than 50% of how what you say is interpreted, and tone of voice is nearly 40%. It's thought that if your words and body cues don't match, only 7% of communication is what you say! So if something is getting in the way of what you want to achieve, don't stand there with your arms crossed, talking in a stern tone of voice while asking for something with supposedly sweet words. The message will get mixed up for sure.

If you have ever seen the Cingular commercial with a mother and daughter shouting at each other, you'll know what I mean. In this ad, a mother hands her daughter a cell phone, and their body language and tone of voice scream conflict. They are moving quickly, their volume is elevated, limbs are flailing, and arms are crossed. But when you listen to what they are saying, they are saying "I love you" and "You never hated me and you never will." It's a brilliant bit of advertising, and exemplifies the dominance of our non-verbal cues. So if someone does something you prefer they didn't and yet you want to respond positively, instead of slamming your hands on your hips, jutting out your neck, and bugging your eyes out in annoyance, take a moment to breathe, keep your hands down, and keep your tone of voice neutral. You'll have access to a much better frame of mind, explaining what went wrong, and the person you are communicating with is much more likely to listen to what you're saying instead of immediately jumping to the defensive. Be aware of your body language and your tone of voice, because unless they're in line with what your words are saying, they will completely change the response you get from the people you are speaking with.

To put a visual on this step in the process, imagine a megaphone held to your mouth, and a camera on your body. Do you want to use that megaphone to get what you want, or to sabotage yourself? Do you want to look at that camera reel and see your body language totally out of sync with what you want to accomplish? We all have the choice about how to use communication, so by being conscious of your body and tone of voice, and by using "I statements," active listening, and the pause, we are much more likely to get the support we want to both raise our children and pursue our goals.

CHAPTER 9
MAKE IT ALL COME TOGETHER

"Be miserable. Or motivate yourself. Whatever has to be done, it's always your choice."

—Wayne Dyer

W hen Sacha came to me, she was a well-educated former professional who had chosen to be a stay-at-home mom. She had waited until later in life to have her children, focusing on her career early in her 20s and 30s, and now that she was lucky enough to have children, she felt it was her duty and privilege to raise them herself. She had anticipated some exhaustion, since the children were still small, but little did she expect the feeling of overwhelming loneliness, resentment, and loss. Her husband had supported her decision to stay at home, but he was confused to see the struggling woman she had become—he wanted her to do what made her happy, and while clearly something wasn't right, neither of them was sure what to do.

After finding the Flex Mom philosophy, circling back with her husband, and working through the steps outlined in this book, Sacha emerged with a renewed sense of passion and excitement about her life. She realized she could still be the primary caregiver for her children, while continuing to pursue her own goals. She doubled down on her support network, renewed her connections with her community, and carved space out of her life to begin writing again. Using the communication skills she learned, she was able to talk with her husband about what she needed from him and what she wanted to create for herself, and their relationship dramatically improved. By extension, her family life felt easier as well, as she involved her children in conversations around her goals and vision for the family. Because she took better care to meet her own needs and make space for her passion, she found she had more energy to focus on the children when they were around.

The Flex Mom is a mom who lives a life somewhere between that of the stay-at-home mom and the working mom. Much like a stay-at-home mom, she is the primary caregiver for her children, but what sets her apart is that she knows how to create the space and implement the structures to pursue her own passions outside the home. The Flex Mom flows between multiple roles, and the energy she gets from being lit up with excitement about pursuing her goals fuels back into her home life.

What do Flex Moms do that sets them apart? They:

- Avoid judgment
- Take care of themselves
- Set clear goals that are in line with their passions
- Redefine their boundaries and community

- Remain mindful about how to be flexible when things inevitably change
- Master skills around communication

It's tough for me to leave you here with just theories about what's needed to make the shift from surviving stay-at-home parenting to thriving in parenthood, without knowing that I've been able to help you make positive changes in your life. I remember slogging through the early stages of stay-at-home parenting, feeling the blows from other people's judgment—and my own harsh judgment of myself—and getting knocked back down the happiness scale. I also know that, as I ruminated on how to make this a better experience for myself and by extension my children, the skills and exercises I used to aid my own transformation into a Flex Mom had a very positive impact on my whole family.

My hope and dream for you, reader, is that you are able to not only understand these theories but also apply them to your lives. If you can't quite figure out how to get there on your own, or if this feels like solving a Rubik's Cube, know that help is out there. You don't have to do this work on your own and, in fact, it is a sign of strength to ask for help when you need it. You can work with a coach, a close friend, your partner, or even join our Flex Mom program. Please don't think that spending time on yourself is selfish because, in all reality, it is probably more selfish to be miserable and secretly blame your unhappiness on someone or something else. If nothing else, be motivated to make these changes for your children—let them see you work on yourself, as they'll see by example that it's okay to follow their passions and invest in themselves.

Lastly, please don't hesitate to reach out and share your success story! I would love to know that you are building on what you're already doing and taking concrete steps to create a thriving Flex Mom life for yourself and your family, because being present with your children is a wonderful gift, and the world could use more happier parents.

BOOK CLUB QUESTIONS

1. What is the significance of the title? Would you have given the book a different title? What would you have called it?
2. What made this book different than other books on the topic of motherhood? Do you think it was better or worse?
3. What was the most memorable part of the book for you? Why did it make an impression? Read your favorite passage of the book out loud and explain what it made you think about.
4. What have you learned from reading this book?
5. How controversial are the issues raised in the book? Who is aligned on which side of the issues, and where you do you fall in the line-up?
6. What surprised you most about the book?
7. Has anything ever happened to you similar to what happened in the book? Did you react in a similar or different manner, and why?

8. Did this book succeed in outlining a different approach to the working mom vs. stay-at-home mom dichotomy? If so, how has it changed your opinion? If not, where did the book fall short?

9. How did the book affect you? Do you feel "changed" in any way?

10. While this book was written with stay-at-home moms in mind, what points are applicable to working moms?

11. What did you find surprising about the facts introduced in this book? For example, multi-tasking, sleep, communication skills…

12. What solutions does the author propose? How probable is the success of implementing those solutions in your life?

FURTHER READING

Books

The Happiness Advantage by Shawn Achor

Happier by Tal Ben-Shahar

NurtureShock by Po Bronson

The 5 Love Languages by Gary Chapman

The Power of Habit by Charles Duhigg

The Secrets of Happy Families by Bruce Feiler

The Desire Map by Danielle LaPorte

Unequal Childhoods: Class, Race, and Family Life by Annette Lareau

Nonverbal Communication by Albert Mehrabian

Take Time for Your Life by Cheryl Richardson

The Instinct to Heal by David Servan-Schreiber

Reclaiming Conversation by Sherry Turkle

The Art of Doing Nothing by Veronique Vienne

Everyday Bliss for Busy Women by Maryam Webster

Skills & Personality Tests

VIA Strengths Survey {free}. URL: http://www.viacharacter.org/www/
Character-Strengths-Survey

Jaime Myers' Body Compass {free}. URL: https://soundcloud.com/
queenmom-1/shine-tribe-body-compass/s-0c480

Myers-Briggs Test online {free}. URL: https://lonerwolf.com/myer-
briggs-free-test/

Myers-Briggs Test, 16 Personalities {free}. URL: https://
www.16personalities.com/free-personality-test

Enneagram Test online {free}. URL: http://www.enneagramcentral.
com/OnlineTest/testa.htm

Fascination Test online {paid}. URL: www.howtofascinate.com

Kolbe Test online {paid}. URL: https://secure.kolbe.com/k2/show_
takeIndex/indexType_A

Clips & References

Cingular—Mother Love advertisement. {Online} URL: https://www.
youtube.com/watch?v=9GQBABkFI34

Manson, M., 2014. 7 Strange Questions that Help You Find Your Life
Purpose. {Online} URL: https://markmanson.net/life-purpose

Misra, S., Cheng, L., Genevie, J., Yuan, M., 2014. The iPhone Effect:
The Quality of In-Person Social Interactions in the Presence of
Mobile Devices. {Online} URL: http://journals.sagepub.com/doi/
abs/10.1177/0013916514539755

Gottman, John, article by Lisitsa, E., 2013. The Four Horsemen:
Contempt {Online} URL: https://www.gottman.com/blog/the-
four-horsemen-contempt/

Mehrabian, A., Wiener, M., 1967. Decoding of inconsistent
communications. {Online} URL: psycnet.apa.org/
psycinfo/1967-08861-001

Mehrabian, A., Ferris, S., 1967. Inference of attitudes from nonverbal communication in two channels. {Online} URL: psycnet.apa.org/psycinfo/1967-10403-001

Crum, A., Langer, E., 2007. Mind-set Matters: Exercise and the placebo effect. {Online} URL: http://nrs.harvard.edu/urn-3:HUL.InstRepos:3196007

Kahneman, D., et al., 2004. A Survey Method for Characterizing Daily Life Experience: The Day Reconstruction Method. {Online} URL: http://www.uvm.edu/pdodds/files/papers/others/everything/kahneman2004a.pdf

Schweizer, T., Kan, K., Hung, Y., Tam, F., Naglie, G., Graham, S., 2013. Brain activity during driving with distraction: an immersive fMRI study. {Online} URL: https://www.ncbi.nlm.nih.gov/pmc/articles/PMC3584251/

Ophir, E., Nass, C., Wagner, A., 2009. Cognitive control in media multitaskers. {Online} URL: http://www.pnas.org/content/106/37/15583.full?sid=5cec06a8-6040-4f12-ad75-07208243ebdc

Employment Characteristics of Families Summary - 2015, from the Bureau of Labor Statistics, released 2016. {Online} URL: https://www.bls.gov/news.release/famee.nr0.htm

Sleep and Sleep Disorders, from Centers for Disease Control and Prevention. About Sleep. {Online} URL: https://www.cdc.gov/sleep/about_sleep/index.html

Sleep.Org powered by the National Sleep Foundation. {Online} URL: https://sleep.org

ACKNOWLEDGEMENTS

I wouldn't be in the world of positive psychology and life coaching if it hadn't been for a chance encounter with an old college instructor. More than seven years after I had sat in his section, and about a month after a friend and I talked about "that teacher who taught me about flow" whose name I couldn't remember, my mom dragged me to a yoga retreat that she felt I had to go on with her. First class in, Tal Ben-Shahar is sitting across from me in the big circle, and I spent the weekend lit up with excitement about the world of wellness that he introduced to me. Thank you, Tal, for remembering me, for letting me move to Cambridge, MA to help teach Positive Psych 1504 under you, for being such a mentor and supporter of mine all these years.

Thank you to Shawn Achor, for trusting me with your name and reputation and continuing to be a supporter and friend, even though it's been years since Cambridge. I deeply admire the life and work you have created, and am so thrilled to see from afar the love you have in your life. Thank you humbly, from the bottom of my heart.

I am grateful to my father who, when he was alive, always reminded me to "keep the balance." I think somewhere in my soul, those words helped me keep moving forward until I found a more balanced, happier way to thrive in the world of parenting.

To my husband, John, for your love, and for knowing me well enough to know when it's the right time for us to jump in with both feet. We just keep getting better. And to my two little wonders, I hope that one day, you understand that I did all of this to be the best mom I could be for you, and that I will make you proud.

To my personal Board of Directors, please know that this book and this movement would not be here today without your unwavering support. Huge thank-you's go to Sarah Bridich for showing me what is possible, and for your many, many hours of conversation and input into this book; Kim Meraz, for your whiteboard sessions and for being the first to tell me I could pull off polka-dotted pedicures; Pagona Xenos, for laughing with me as I broke the massage table and for being a constant source of love and sparkle; Tricia Harrison for walking the highs and lows of motherhood with me, and holding my heart through it all; Jaime Myers for being open to all levels of conversation from spirits to the playground, and for teaching me so much about femininity; Misasha Graham for seeing beyond my college fashion sense and forging a lifetime of sisterhood. To my many other girlfriends and fellow moms who chimed in with contributions or even just nodded yes in support of this idea, thank you. You kept me motivated to craft a book and way of thinking that I hope will help others just like us.

I've been fortunate to stumble onto the path of the Author Incubator, and am ever so grateful that Angela Lauria and her team held my hand through the process of birthing what was simply an idea to the launch of the Flex Mom movement. Thank you for your bluntness, your challenges, your insightful pushes to make this better. This idea for sure would have floundered in my brain, unshared, without your guidance—I have learned so much from you. To my editor Cynthia Kane, thank you for your enthusiastic support and critical eye; this wouldn't be the work it is without you.

To the Morgan James Publishing team: Special thanks to David Hancock, CEO & Founder for believing in me and my message. To my Author Relations Manager, Margo Toulouse, thanks for making the process seamless and easy. Many more thanks to everyone else, but especially Jim Howard, Bethany Marshall, and Nickcole Watkins.

To you, my reader, thank you for picking up a copy of this book! Huge appreciation and kudos for believing in yourself enough to read through this new approach to motherhood. What happens next is up to you, but I hope you choose to claim the title, to step into your role as a Flex Mom, because it's right here for you to be. Our children could use happier mothers, mothers who unleash their amazing, powerful passions to the world.

ABOUT THE AUTHOR

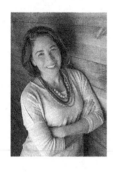 Much like laundry, Sara Blanchard's life runs in cycles. After graduating from Harvard, the financial cycle took her to Tokyo, Hong Kong, and New York. The wellness cycle trained her in life coaching and positive psychology. The parenting cycle—not a cycle, more commitment, call it permanent press— saw her struggling as a stay-at-home mom until she found a better way and founded the Flex Mom movement. On the heels of this book, she has launched a Flex Mom program to help support mothers who wish to clear enough space to pursue their passions while continuing to be the primary caregivers for their children. Sara and her family call Denver home.

Website: http://www.flexmombook.com/

Email: sara@flexmombook.com

Facebook: https://www.facebook.com/sarablanchardauthor/

THANK YOU

Thank you for reading *Flex Mom*! This isn't the end of the journey, but just the beginning of the process of creating a new model of motherhood. I hope this book has given you the tools and confidence to carve out space to pursue your own passions while you continue to be the primary caregiver to your children.

As a Flex Mom in transformation, here is a bonus for you: **A FREE WORKBOOK!**

You can use a copy of this workbook to keep you on track as you move through the Flex Mom process. Included in the pages are placeholders to jot down your strengths and traits, guides for adding to your healthy habits, and space to let your big dreams run free. You can access this workbook at www.flexmombook.com.

Good luck, and keep on making a positive difference in your world.

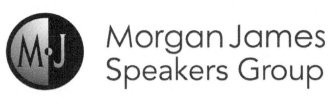

Morgan James
Speakers Group

We connect Morgan James published authors with live and online events and audiences whom will benefit from their expertise.

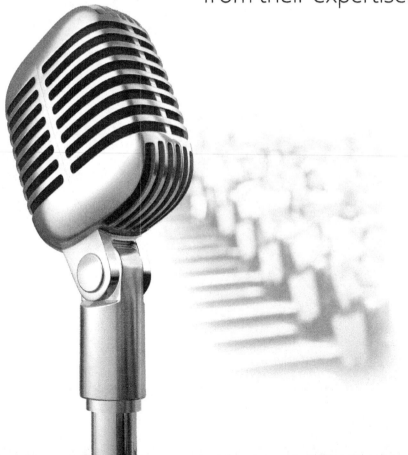

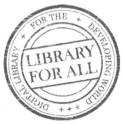

Morgan James makes all of our titles available
through the Library for All Charity Organization.

www.LibraryForAll.org

CPSIA information can be obtained
at www.ICGtesting.com
Printed in the USA
BVOW06s0557020218
507072BV00001B/7/P